Frank G. Addleman, a nutrition and health instructor at Santa Ana Community College in California, is a member of the American College of Sports Medicine, the Nutrition Today Society, and the Society for Nutritional Education.

Prentice-Hall International, Inc., *London*
Prentice-Hall of Australia Pty. Limited, *Sydney*
Prentice-Hall Canada Inc., *Toronto*
Prentice-Hall of India Private Limited, *New Delhi*
Prentic-Hall of Japan, Inc., *Tokyo*
Prentice-Hall of Southeast Asia Pte. Ltd., *Singapore*
Whitehall Books Limited, *Wellington, New Zealand*
Editora Prentice-Hall do Brasil Ltda., *Rio de Janeiro*

THE
WINNING EDGE
Nutrition for Athletic Fitness and Performance

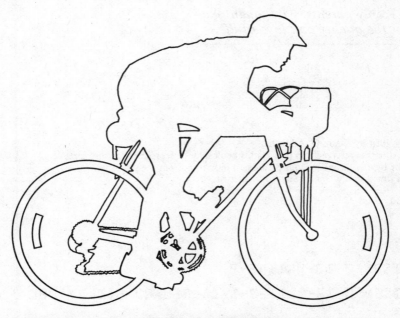

Frank G. Addleman

Prentice-Hall, Inc., Englewood Cliffs, New Jersey 07632

Library of Congress Cataloging in Publication Data

Addleman, Frank G.
  The winning edge.

  Includes index.
  1. Nutrition.   2. Health.   3. Physical fitness—
Nutritional aspects.   1. Title.
QP141.A37   1984   613.2   83-13785
ISBN 0-13-961145-2
ISBN 0-13-961137-1 (A Reward book : pbk.)

*To my parents, who taught me
the quality and love of life.*

10 9 8 7 6 5 4 3 2 1

ISBN 0-13-961145-2

ISBN 0-13-961137-1 (A REWARD BOOK : PBK.)

Editorial/production supervision by Chris McMorrow
Cover design © 1984 by Jeannette Jacobs
Manufacturing buyer: Pat Mahoney

This book is available at a special discount when ordered in
bulk quantities. Contact Prentice-Hall, Inc., General
Publishing Division, Special Sales, Englewood Cliffs, N.J. 07632.

CONTENTS

PREFACE

If you have been confused about the food you eat and its effect on your health, then this book is for you. Using simple and easy-to-understand language, this book cuts through the technical and sophisticated concepts of nutritional science and makes nutrition more meaningful and applicable to you personally.

You will learn the basic functions and roles of the major nutrients—fats, proteins, carbohydrates, vitamins, minerals, and water. You will discover that the proper selection of these nutrients in the form of food not only can contribute to the prevention of diseases, such as cancer and heart disease, but also can enhance or limit your ability to turn in an optimum physical performance.

For the athlete or casual jogger, I have drawn heavily from research in sports physiology. Although I cannot guarantee that good nutrition will make you a champion, I am quite sure that poor nutrition will prevent you from performing at your optimal level. You will discover that through proper food selection you can control both your physical and mental energy levels. You will understand more clearly the effects that each of the nutrients plays not only in preparing you for competition but also in helping you through that competition.

At the end of each chapter, I have included a section for questions and answers. This approach will help clarify each of the areas discussed. I think you will find them very informative.

The subject of weight control gets extra consideration in this book. Because weight control is almost a national pastime, it is appropriate to cover the subject in some detail. Weight control can be a major factor in your health as well as in your performance. You not only will learn the dangers of low-calorie crash diets, but you will discover that they may even make you fatter! Some of the new theories of how we use energy will be discussed, and you will find that diet alone may not be the answer to permanent weight control.

Rather than suggest that athletes eat like everyone else, I think that we should all eat like athletes. Activity and proper nutrition should go hand in hand in our quest for total health. After reading this book you will have a much better understanding of the food you eat. If you put that knowledge to proper use, you will have laid the foundation for better health and performance.

This book is the result of many years of teaching nutrition. It would not have materialized without the encouragement of many students, friends, and athletes. Many people took part in the actual production of the manuscript. I would like to thank them all, along with special thanks to Dennis Fawcett of Prentice-Hall, who accepted this manuscript for publication. Last, but not least, I thank my wife, Betty, for her patience and encouragement during the writing of this book.

1

NUTRITION:
THE LINK TO HEALTH
AND PERFORMANCE

Many facets of health, ranging from physical fitness and stress control to our individual genetic makeups, have been cited as the keys to health and performance. Even though each of these factors plays a major role in total health, a considerable amount of scientific evidence indicates that nutrition is the main environmental factor within our control that affects our health. As a society Americans are bombarded with advertising and fad diets that promise to make us younger, sexier, faster, trimmer, and stronger. Our choices run the gamut from high-protein diets that promise trim bodies or big muscles to vegetarian diets that separate foods into "yin" and "yang," implying that certain foods yield beneficial powers and that some are adverse to good health. Recently, diet has even become the cause for alarm as we hear that almost everything we eat causes either cancer, heart disease, or some equally debilitating disease. We might wonder how we survived over the centuries without the aid of special diets, vitamin and mineral supplements, and all the "wonder foods" we have today. With all this conflicting information it is no wonder that most Americans are totally confused about what to eat.

Our Changing Diet

Our diet, like the rest of the environment, has undergone considerable change since primitive times. Primitive people didn't have the luxury (or distraction) of all the food choices we are offered today. If they wanted meat on the table it meant hunting for wild game rather than dropping in at a hamburger stand. When their sweet tooth increased their desire for sugar, they didn't have the convenience of a soft drink or a candy bar. They had to make do with fresh fruit or some other natural carbohydrate. Simply put, it was difficult for people to make poor nutritional choices since the food selection available to them was natural, wholesome, and sufficient for their physiological needs.

The problem is much different today. The natural foods that we have survived on for millions of years are still available to us but, because of food technology, our choices have changed. In a sense, we have been taken out of our natural food environment and placed in an environment that allows us to make many different food choices. Our choices are no longer based on natural instinct but, rather on advertising, convenience, and taste. Take sweets as an example. If you are hungry your body encourages you to eat. If you are at work and only have a ten-minute break, it's *convenient* to get a cola and pastry from the vending machine. It also tastes good. Advertising plays a role because we subconsciously remember ads telling us that sugar foods give us quick energy. Our primitive friend had to settle for a nutritious apple! We make other, less conspicuous, selections, too. Take, for example, eggs. We have heard that they are high in cholesterol and that cholesterol is associated with heart disease. We have also heard that eggs are a very nutritious food, and we know that people have been eating eggs for hundreds of years. That's true, but look how easy it is for us to go to the market and buy two dozen eggs. Our primitive friends had to chase down wild game or raid nests to collect their eggs. Who do you think ends up eating too many eggs? We hear that cereal is a good alternative to bacon and eggs for breakfast every day, but if we don't know the good ones from the bad ones we end up making some poor selections. Many of the cereals available have too much added refined sugar, and in excess that can be bad for your health. A final example: When was the last time you sat down to dinner with the family and ate a meal cooked from scratch? A long time ago, right? In fact, the last meal you all ate together was probably a "Chicken Delight" take-out dinner for six at the *convenient* price of $3.99 each.

The problem is obvious. There are so many poor food choices available that are convenient and cheap that it seems burdensome to take the time to select food that is more nutritious and takes more of our precious time to prepare. But all is not lost. With some basic understanding of nutrition we can easily swing the pendulum to a more nutritious diet and increase our state of health and performance.

Nutrition and Disease

A common misconception about nutrition is that people who attempt to improve their diets are "health freaks" seeking a utopia of well-being, whereas the rest of us maintain perfectly good health with little or no concern about what we eat. Nutritionists may not know for sure what the ideal diet is, but there is little disagreement among them that the American diet is not conducive to good health. There is an old American saying: "Eat all your food, people are starving all over the world." The maxim in today's underdeveloped countries might be "Eat all your rice, Americans are starving on junk food."

People become ill, suffer disability, and even die prematurely simply because of the way they live. There is mounting scientific evidence that the way we live our lives is the major determinant not only of how long but of how well we live. The new era in health will take us beyond traditional medical care and stop illness before it occurs through personal prevention and the promotion of healthy life-styles.

Diet, the major element of life-style, is strongly linked to the incidence of degenerative diseases in this country. Cardiovascular disease, which includes heart disease and stroke, is most commonly associated with diet. Vascular diseases account for over half the deaths in the United States, a fact directly related to our typical high-fat diet. Obesity, a disease that is the underlying cause of many other diseases such as hypertension and age-onset diabetes, starts with the problem of weight control. The constant battle to control weight, which seems to occupy many Americans, is rooted in our excessive intake of processed foods high in fat, refined sugar, and empty calories. Other diseases, such as breast cancer, colon cancer, osteoporosis, hypoglycemia, and tooth decay, are all significantly more prevalent in people who eat the typical American diet.

Nutrition and Performance

Humans are creatures of habit. One of our worst habits—always looking for an easier way—causes dieters to use diet pills to shed unwanted weight and often spurs athletes to look at special foods or supplements to make them champions. In the following chapters there will be no mention of a "wonder food" that will propel the athlete into the championships. Instead, I will show that negative nutrition prevents athletes from reaching their potential and that positive nutrition enhances that potential. Nutrition is an important link to success and should be treated as such. Great athletes in any sport must start with great talent. Given that basic gift, they must have the desire and dedication to excel in their particular sport. From there, it is hard training, drilling, and self-discipline that produces champions. Positive nutrition will enhance total training and performance, while negative nutrition will probably prevent the athlete from reaching his or her ultimate goal. Athletes and coaches often miss this important link. They frequently feel that training is the only factor and that nutrition has little effect. That is a logical assumption, especially when athletes appear to perform successfully on a "normal" diet. There is no question that highly gifted athletes can, on certain occasions, perform well in spite of a poor diet. But they will never reach their maximum potential.

A Champion or an Also-Ran

We constantly hear that athletes should eat just like everyone else except for consuming more calories, which are required for their increased energy expenditures. That view is not totally correct because it is based on the assumption that everyone else eats a good diet, and we know that's not the case. If, in fact, athletes are eating like everyone else, then we can assume we can really increase our performance if we break away from the group, so to speak, and eat a more nutritious diet. In fact, that's exactly what can happen.

I have witnessed an amazing number of athletes fail in their final effort because of poor nutrition. They seem to forget that if the average person can fall victim to illness and fail to perform at an optimum level, the same thing can happen to them. If you're going to demand an optimum performance, then you're going to have to supply optimum fuel, and you're not going to get that on the typical diet, which has been shown to be unhealthy. Neither will it come from the haphazard use of supplements, strength pills, endurance pills, or some other miracle food that you simply add to your already poor diet. Optimum performance will result from a total balancing of your nutritional requirements, and it will take as much thought and concern as you put into the other aspects of your training program.

Many coaches and athletes have a hard time seeing this relationship between nutrition and winning. It's obvious to them that increased strength is related to increased performance, so weight training is needed. An athlete would scoff at anyone who suggested that it's not important to train at a high level or to perfect his or her techniques. What isn't so obvious is that positive nutrition *enhances every factor essential to winning!* Athletes may be seriously damaging their performance by ignoring this fact. They fail to change their diets because the benefits of good nutrition are not as tangible as the results of conditioning and training. It is simply not obvious that nutrition plays a major role in condition and affects both physical and psychological responses.

5

Although we often see athletes defeat themselves through poor dietary habits, we seldom see this occur in the training of racehorses. Their diet, just like their training, is controlled. Their trainers make sure that the animals eat a balance of the correct nutrients in the form of grains, alfalfa, and vitamin and mineral preparations.

It's very obvious to most people that animals must receive highly nutritious food. Yet these same people think that they can survive quite well on junk! No one would feed a dog soda, potato chips, hot dogs, or ice cream. When athletes start thinking of themselves and feeding themselves as thoroughbreds, they will see an improvement in total performance that will extend over a lifetime.

Nutrition can be our weak link, or it can enhance every aspect of training. With proper nutrition our energy level and enthusiasm will increase and our overall ability to perform will improve. A good diet helps make champion athletes and improves performance.

THE EFFECTS
OF POSITIVE NUTRITION
ON ATHLETIC PERFORMANCE

Increased energy level

Increased energy reserves

Increased mental alertness

Ability to train at higher levels

Increased fitness level

Ability to handle higher levels of stress

Increased strength

Increased available training time due to a decrease in time lost from colds, infection, and illness

Rapid rehabilitation from injuries and illness

Maintenance of ideal weight

Decrease in excess body fat

Increase in muscle mass

Positive psychological attitude toward training and competition

A Better Diet for Health

Research into the effects of diet on health has taken scientists around the world in search of the ideal diet. They have discovered entire peoples in Russia, the Himalayas, Ecuador, and Mexico with diets and life-styles quite different from ours, all of whom seem to have in common an astonishing lack of the degenerative diseases common in industrialized nations. These people live long, healthy, active lives. Of course, other factors besides nutrition play a role in their health and longevity. They usually live at high altitudes where the air is free from smog and the water is pure and free from chemicals. Most are farmers working rugged land. They are spared the stresses of industrialized societies, and they get plenty of exercise from work as well as from recreation.

An exceptional example is that of the Tarahumarha Indians of Mexico, who play a recreational game involving kicking a wooden ball for more than 100 miles. This grueling activity is performed over rugged terrain and resembles soccer in that team members kick the ball back and forth to one another as they run. Their diet consists mostly of plant food with a limited amount of animal products. They are not exposed to processed foods, which are highly adulterated with fats and sugar. Obesity, heart disease, and diabetes are all nonexistent in their cultures. To be sure, they don't have the conveniences of modern housing, sanitation, and medical services, yet they are healthy and alert. Obviously, we are unlikely to drop everything and move to the Andes or join the Tarahumarha Indians in kickball. However, we can learn to incorporate those aspects of their life-style which contribute to their good health into our modern life-style. We need to get back on the track because we have let all the conveniences of a technological society steal one of our most precious national assets: our health and well-being.

Even our own government has begun to recognize the health problems related to our diet. In 1977, the Senate Select Committee on Nutrition was formed to evaluate all of the research and to listen to expert testimony relating the American diet to disease. The evidence associating our eating patterns with disease was very impressive. But association and circumstantial evidence are not direct proof that diet causes or prevents disease. Naturally, the powerful lobbyists of the giant food conglomerates were quick to point this out. They are well aware that if they can show one shred of evidence disproving the link between their products and disease, a nutritionally uneducated public will probably choose to ignore all the other facts. So far these tactics seem to have worked very well. Processed-food sales are up—not down!

There are several general diet changes you can make to improve your health and performance and decrease your exposure to disease:

FATS: We all eat too much fat. Average Americans consume 42% of their calories in fat. We should reduce this to 30% or less. Only 10% of our total calories should be eaten in the form of saturated fats.

CHOLESTEROL: We should consume about 300 milligrams a day or less.

CARBOHYDRATES: We presently eat only 28% of our calories in the form of complex carbohydrates. We should increase that amount to at least 48%.

SUGAR: We eat twice as much refined and processed sugar as we should. Refined and processed sugar should account for no more than 10% of our total calorie intake.

SALT: The average person consumes too much salt, in some cases as many as 20 grams a day or more (about 4 teaspoons). We should reduce this to fewer than 5 grams a day. We can get by very well on about 1/10 teaspoon.

PROTEIN: Many of us eat more than we require, and we eat too much protein from expensive animal sources.

EXERCISE: Most Americans do not exercise enough. We should exercise regularly to control our weight and increase our cardiovascular fitness.

TOBACCO, ALCOHOL, AND DRUGS: True health will not occur if we abuse the use of tobacco, alcohol, and drugs.

Learning about Good Nutrition

Learning about good nutrition in today's marketplace is no easy task. It's easy to tell someone to reduce his or her cholesterol intake, but that doesn't mean just substituting margarine for butter or using more vegetable oil, in spite of what the advertisements say. The food industry is way ahead of nutritionists in telling the public what is healthy, but they often don't tell the whole story. They sell margarine, which is cholesterol-free, but switching from butter to margarine won't do a thing for the eater's total fat intake or, for that matter, for the cholesterol intake. Just going from one fat to the other misses the whole point that all fat intake should be reduced.

Other terms, like *complex carbohydrates, refined sugar, saturated fat,* and *polyunsaturated fat,* are very confusing to the average person. Take salt, for example. A student of mine assumed that he was not eating a lot of salt simply because he didn't salt his food. He was unaware that the majority of our salt intake comes from processed foods, which have salt *added.* You're lucky if you can find a food product made that doesn't have added salt.

In the following chapters, the field of nutrition is explained in the simplest terms. You will be able to understand a science that has become more complex for the average person, and, more importantly, you will be able to apply it to your daily eating habits. The result of following a positive nutritional program will be an increase in your health and performance.

Questions and Answers

Q: *Every time I read about a diet it says it might increase my life by from five to ten years. Maybe that's not worth it to me. What do you think?*
A: I think you want to have your cake and eat it too! No one can give you any guarantees of a longer life or a life with more quality, but I would feel pretty safe in saying that chances for serious disease and early death will be greatly increased if you have a

poor diet, don't exercise, smoke, etc. I remember seeing a film on cancer in which a woman who had smoked for twenty years was dying of cancer. She said she didn't care if she died ten years earlier at 65 instead of 75. She thought the ten years was taken off the end, not the middle! She died of lung cancer soon after reaching forty years of age.

Q: *My grandfather is sixty years old. He has a terrible diet, doesn't exercise, and smokes. How did he make it?*
A: I can't attest to the quality of his life, but if he's really healthy, which I doubt, he's an exception to the rule. Most sixty-year-old men in the United States have many ailments, lack energy, and suffer some advanced degree of circulatory disease. Being alive as opposed to being dead is not a measurement of one's state of health!

Q: *Don't most of us buy what we want? No one forces us to buy a product.*
A: Big Brother is here! McDonald's alone spends $120 million a year in advertising telling you what to eat. You have to go out of your way to eat right today, because most of the time the easiest choice is a poor one. How many times have you had fries, a milkshake, and a hamburger because they were fast, cheap, and convenient? If you just follow your taste buds in today's highly processed food market, you'll be in real trouble. We must learn to shut our eyes and ears to the advertising.

Q: *Can you give me other examples of how my food dollar is controlled by industry and not by me?*
A: Yes. You don't see ads for skim or nonfat milk, do you? Only "milk" is advertised, and if they promoted the wholesome nonfat milk, what would they do with all that fat? How often do you see ads for whole-grain breads and cereals? Not too often; but you see plenty of ads aimed at children, promoting sugared cereals, candy, pastries, and other junk foods. Come to think of it, maybe your child has become an agent for the food industry and tells you what to spend your money on! Do you seriously think your great-grandmother would consciously walk into a supermarket and say, "Give me a box of your sugar-coated green and yellow

breakfast cereal"? Such an act is learned behavior, not intelligent choice.

Q: *How do we eat differently from our grandparents?*
A: We eat more processed and convenience foods, such as instant dinners, instant breakfast drinks, and packaged and canned products. Although not all of them are bad, they are usually excessive in sugar, fat, and calories, and are low in nutrients and fiber. Because both husband and wife are working in more families, we eat out more. One-third of our food dollar is spent on fast foods, many of which are high in sugar, fat, protein, and calories, the very things we should reduce in our diet.

Q: *Will improved nutrition really have that much effect on my health?*
A: That really depends on how bad your diet is now. The more deficient the diet, the more marked the improvement will be. Nutrition is a major component of total health, but to develop optimum health, a person must evaluate all of his or her health habits, including exercise, smoking, and stress control.

Q: *Teen-agers, especially athletes, seem so trim and healthy, yet they eat all kinds of junk. Why don't they experience disease?*
A: Many do. Obesity and overweight are very characteristic problems among teen-agers. For a simple answer to your question, look at an ex-athlete at forty years of age. Get the picture? Degeneration takes many years, and if teen-agers continue a life-style of nutritional abuses, they will suffer the same illnesses and diseases as their parents. I often ask students if they would like to have the same state of health when they are older that their parents have now. They look at me and shake their heads—No!

Q: *When I eat a poor diet and then switch to a good diet for a few days, I still feel the same.*
A: You are taught to expect instant results, but things just don't happen that way. You get fat very slowly—it often takes years—but you expect to lose it all in two weeks. I'm sure that if you smoked a cigarette and woke up the next day with lung cancer, it wouldn't take long for you to quit smoking. Attempt to change

your eating habits at a rate that will assure some long-term changes, and you will begin to experience a better state of health.

Q: *Are all those diseases you listed the result of eating wrong?*
A: Diet surely has the strongest link to most of them, but it's not always the direct cause. Heredity can predispose some of us to certain diseases in spite of our precautions. Other factors, such as our level of exercise, exposure to chemicals, stress, and use of alcohol, have an impact on our chances of developing certain diseases.

Q: *As a coach I can't see where diet can have much effect on performance. How much does it have?*
A: It's relative. I might ask the same question about conditioning, weight training, or drills. I know of many athletes who weight train all the time but still don't win. That doesn't mean weight training is unimportant. You have to analyze the whole program and then see where you can enhance it. Positive nutrition enables an athlete to derive the maximum benefits from training.

Q: *I've seen athletes on all kinds of bizarre diets and supplements. They seem to swear by them, but I don't see them performing better than the athletes who ignore their diets.*
A: Athletes are a superstitious breed. They'll try anything to win. Bizarre diets and unlimited use of supplements are hardly scientific approaches to improved performance. They may help, purely by accident, but they also may be a hindrance. Ignoring diet altogether can be just as bad. If you're performing well on a poor diet, imagine what you might do on a good diet! If a miler smokes and still runs the mile in 4:10 minutes, should he or she continue to smoke?

Q: *It seems that athletes have been getting along fine for years without any concern for diet. Why all the concern?*
A: There was a time when football players got along fine without weight training! When players became stronger from lifting weights, everyone got on the bandwagon or they were left behind. Look for the weak link to success and then improve it. For most athletes nutrition is that weak link.

Q: *There is not much you can do if you have a genetic weakness for a disease, is there?*
A: Yes. A genetic weakness simply means you have a greater chance of getting a certain disease. A person at risk should choose a life-style to reduce the risk. For example, if your doctor says you have a strong history of heart disease in your family, you are not necessarily going to get heart disease. But you had better pay more attention to the risk factors—and what you eat is a major risk factor!

Q: *What if I ignore all of your suggestions?*
A: Visit a few hospitals and homes for the elderly so you can get an idea of what your future holds. Carry a large insurance policy. Buy a cemetery plot. Don't, by any means, plan for the future. Be a fatalist, and you are guaranteed the same life as the typical American. Welcome to the diet cola generation!

Q: *Will I see a direct effect on my performance from eating a better diet?*
A: That depends on how bad it is now. In time you will notice your level of training will improve, which in turn will result in an improved performance. Don't just measure the success of your diet by performance. The long-range benefits of better health will be equally important later in life.

2
FATS: EATING LESS FOR BETTER HEALTH

Fats and Their Function

Body fat and dietary fat are often confusing factors in any discussion of fat. Body fat doesn't come just from eating too much fat. Fat can be manufactured from carbohydrates and protein, especially if you eat too many calories of these nutrients. A reasonable amount of body fat is essential to good health. It gives insulation to the body, cushions internal organs, supplies oils in your skin, and is part of hormone substances in cell membranes.

Dietary fat supplies the essential fatty acid linoleic acid from which the body can manufacture all the other fats essential to health. Fats must contribute only a small percentage of your total calorie intake, about 3%, for good health. The main sources of this essential fat are whole grains, vegetables, and nuts. The polyunsaturated oils such as corn oil and safflower oil are excellent sources as well. These dietary fats supply a concentrated source of energy and transport the fat-soluble vitamins A, D, E, and K through the digestive tract. Saturated fats, which are found in abundance in animal products, are actually not required by the human body. Unfortunately, they are the fats that we consume in excess, and there is strong evidence that they do a lot of damage to our health.

Fats and Disease

The present circumstantial evidence shows a strong correlation between a high-fat, high-cholesterol diet and heart disease and cancer. It is not the only correlation. Other factors, such as smoking, high blood pressure, lack of exercise, stress, vitamin and mineral deficiency, and excess use of refined sugars, have all been linked to these diseases.

ATHEROSCLEROSIS

Atherosclerosis is a disease of the arteries that is characterized by progressive thickening and hardening of the artery walls. This leads to arterial occlusion (narrowing of the artery diameter), which reduces the amount of oxygen and nutrients available to the cells of body. The coronary arteries, which feed the heart, are particularly susceptible to this narrowing. Total closure can cause a heart attack. A stroke, which is a loss of blood supply to the brain, can occur as a result of occlusion of the blood vessels that supply oxygen and nutrients to the brain. Cholesterol, a fat-like substance found in all animal products and a few plant products, is the major substance that accumulates on the artery walls and causes the progressive narrowing of the arteries. Dietary fats, especially saturated fats, seem to increase this accumulation of cholesterol on the artery walls.

Atherosclerosis accounts for about half of the deaths in the United States. It seems that every time you hear or read about someone dying it's from a heart attack, stroke, or other vascular disease. Most of these are the result of arterial occlusion. Much of the evidence around the world indicates that populations that eat a high-fat and high-cholesterol diet have significantly more deaths from coronary disease. Finland, the country which has the highest fat intake, also has the highest death rate from coronary disease. Japan, on the other hand, has a very low death rate from coronary diseases, and its citizens consume a very low-fat diet.

WHAT IS CHOLESTEROL?

Most people assume that cholesterol is a fat because we are told to eat less fat to lower our cholesterol level. Actually, cholesterol is a sterol, a complicated almost waxlike substance found only in animal products. Although the body uses it in cell walls and in the manufacture of vitamin D and some hormones, it is probable that we can function quite well without any cholesterol in the diet. Our bodies are capable of manufacturing all the cholesterol they need for good health.

Cholesterol blood level tests are recorded in milligrams of cholesterol per 100 milliliters of serum. The general rule is that the higher the cholesterol level, the higher the potential for heart disease. There is, however, still disagreement over where to place the acceptable level. Heart specialists, however, generally prefer a low level—200 milligrams or less.

There is some evidence to suggest that a cholesterol count of 150 milligrams or less is a sound preventive measure, since it appears that people with readings this low experience a very low incidence of heart disease.

Several studies, including the famous Framingham study (a study that started in 1949 and continued for 24 years to examine the lifestyles and health of six thousand men and women in Framingham, Massachusettes), have shown that the risk of coronary disease is five times as great for men thirty-five to forty-five years of age who have cholesterol levels above 260 milligrams per 100 milliliters of serum, as compared to men whose cholesterol levels are below 200.

Since the average dietary intake in our country is around 600 milligrams of cholesterol a day, with atheletes who consume enormous amounts of meat and dairy products taking in well over 1,000 milligrams, it is apparent that as a society we need to greatly reduce the amount of cholesterol we eat. Most experts recommend a daily intake of less than 300 milligrams a day.

CHOLESTEROL CONTENT OF ANIMAL PRODUCTS
IN MILLIGRAMS (mg.) (Approximate)

MEAT (1 OUNCE)

Brains	— 600 mg.	Veal	— 30 mg.
Kidney	— 225 mg.	Pork, Lamb, Beef	— 30 mg.
Liver	— 125 mg.		

DAIRY

Whole Milk	—	35 mg.	— 1 cup
Skim Milk	—	6 mg.	— 1 cup
Creamed Cottage Cheese	—	50 mg.	— 1 cup
Uncreamed Cottage Cheese	—	15 mg.	— 1 cup
Cream	—	60 mg.	— 3 ounces
Ice Cream	—	60 mg.	— 1 cup
Cheese	—	30 mg.	— 1 ounce
Egg Yolk	—	250 mg.	— 1 egg

SEAFOOD (1 OUNCE)

Shrimp	— 40 mg.	Tuna	— 18 mg.
Crab	— 30 mg.	Halibut	— 12 mg.
Lobster	— 25 mg.	Salmon	— 12 mg.
Clams	— 18 mg.	Oysters	— 12 mg.

FOWL

Chicken/Turkey:	Light Meat	— 22 mg.	— 1 ounce
	Dark Meat	— 25 mg.	— 1 ounce

FATS

Butter	— 35 mg.	— 1 tablespoon
Lard	— 12 mg.	— 1 tablespoon

CANCER

According to Dr. Frank Rhuscher, Jr., senior vice-president of research for the American Cancer Society, "The A.C.S. is getting awfully close to the point of condemning high-fat diets as a major cancer risk factor." Epidemiological studies show a low incidence of many types of cancer when the diet is low in fat. For example, the Japanese, who traditionally eat a low-fat diet, have a very low incidence of breast and colon cancer. In cultures where the fat intake is high, cancer, especially breast and colon cancer, is more prevalent. There is also evidence that when the diet is high in polyunsaturated oils, the link with cancer may be strongest. Although the facts are not yet conclusive and the reasons for the link are not yet clear, the probability that fats may increase our risk of cancer and heart disease is a strong reason to dramatically lower fat intake.

TISSUE ANOXIA

Anoxia is a lack of oxygen to the cells. Repeated studies have shown that a high-fat diet can reduce the available oxygen in the blood reaching the cells. Once in the blood system, fats cause the red blood cells, which carry oxygen, to clump together, thus decreasing circulation through the small capillaries of the body. It is also suspected that this reduction in available oxygen could be a contributing factor in coronary insufficiency and anginal pain experienced by heart patients. The important findings with regard to this issue were brought to light by Dr. Myer Friedman, Study Director for the National Heart, Lung, and Blood Institute.

PLATELET CLUMPING
AND ARTERY SPASM

A recent study by Dr. Dean Ornish from the Baylor College of Medicine, Houston, Texas, appeared in the *Journal of the American Medical Association*. This study, which dealt with the effects of diet and emotional stress, pointed out that a high fat diet not only contributed to atherosclerosis (progressive build up of plaque on the artery walls) but can cause platelet clumping and artery spasm. Platelet clumping is actually blood clotting, which is fine if you have a cut, but when it occurs in the coronary arteries it reduces the available oxygen to the heart and can contribute to sudden death. Artery spasm does much the same thing by contracting the smooth muscle lining of the arteries thus reducing or closing off the oxygen supply to the heart. Other factors such as stress and smoking can also trigger platelet clumping and artery spasm.

OBESITY AND FAT

Considering the average American's diet, it is not surprising that so many people in this country face an excess-weight problem at some time in their lives. Most people think that carbohydrates (bread, potatoes, etc.) cause the overweight problem. Actually, it's fat that makes us fat! Specifically, it is the dietary fat we consume in our food. Milk is a good example of wasted fat calories. An 8-ounce glass of whole milk contains 170 calories, of which 90 calories are fat. If that same 8-ounce glass contained skim milk, it would have only 90 calories and no fat. In other words, by removing the fat we save calories but still get to drink eight ounces of milk. Who said we have to eat less to lose weight?

Maintaining an ideal weight makes us feel better and improves our self-image. But more importantly, excess weight, especially when it reaches the point of obesity, predisposes us to many diseases. Heart and circulatory diseases and diabetes are the major risk factors of overweight. However, obesity has also been related to low energy, stress, skeletal problems, and hormonal disorders. The best first step in adjusting the diet for weight loss is to reduce the fat consumption.

Understanding Dietary Fats

We primarily should be concerned with understanding saturated and polyunsaturated fats. Many people assume that animal fats, like butter, are saturated fats, while vegetable oils, like safflower oil, are polyunsaturated. Actually, butter has considerably more saturated fat than polyunsaturated fat and safflower oil has more polyunsaturated than saturated, but both are a mixture.

SATURATED FATS

Saturated fat tends to elevate the cholesterol level of the blood, increasing the risk of heart disease. Chemically, in a saturated fat each carbon atom bond holds a hydrogen atom. Saturated fat is like sponge that is holding all the water possible. It is totally saturated. In the case of the fat, however, the saturation is with hydrogen atoms instead of water. As a rule of thumb, the more saturated fat is, the more solid it is at room temperature. Butter and bacon grease are solid at room temperature, an obvious tip-off that they are highly saturated fats. Generally speaking, all animal products are higher in saturated fat than are plant foods.

POLYUNSATURATED FATS

Polyunsaturated fats do not raise the cholesterol level. In fact, they can contribute to lowering it. An oil is said to be more polyunsaturated if it is liquid at room temperature. Using the sponge example again, a polyunsaturated sponge would hold less water. It is not saturated. Two or more of the bonds of the carbon atom are not holding hydrogen. Plant oils are much higher in polyunsaturated fats than animal fats.

HYDROGENATED FATS

So far, fats seem simple to understand. Animal fats are high in saturated fats, and vegetable oils are high in unsaturated fats.

Now for the catch! Food processors love to play with nature. They take polyunsaturated oil, which doesn't raise our cholesterol level, and change it to a saturated fat that does raise our cholesterol level! How? They just fill up the carbon bonds with hydrogen, thus the term "hydrogenated fats." Hydrogenation is the reason margarine, made from vegetable oil, stays hard at room temperature. Why do they hydrogenate it? It's pretty difficult to spread vegetable oil on a piece of bread!

Hydrogenated fats aren't much better than saturated fats. They may even turn out to be dangerous, so they should not be used as substitutes. Avoiding them necessitates your reading the labels on processed foods to see if the vegetable oil used is hydrogenated or not.

We all remember (if we're old enough!) when the oil in a jar of peanut butter filtered to the top. We had to mix it before spreading it on our bread. Most processors hydrogenate peanut butter today, so that the oil won't filter to the top. This makes it more convenient to spread, since it's now smooth and creamy, but it doesn't do the heart much good!

Some typical hydrogenated products are: margarines, processed peanut butter, dairy creamers, imitation dairy products, crackers, and processed nuts.

Reducing Fats and Cholesterol

Generally speaking, we want to reduce our intake of all animal products because they are high in saturated fats and are our only source of dietary cholesterol. Our polyunsaturated fats should come from whole grains, fruits, and vegetables in their least processed state. Oils, such as safflower oil and corn oil, also supply polyunsaturated fats, but because of their high concentration they can easily increase your total dietary fat level too much. They are also very high in calories.

Since the *average* intake of fat in the United States provides 42% of our total calories, it's logical to assume that many Americans consume much more. The recommendations for reducing our fat intake range from limiting it to 35% of total calories, recommended by the American Heart Association, to limiting it to 10% of total calories, recommended on the Spartan Pritikin diet promoted by Nathan Pritikin. This low amount suggested by Pritikin is safe but it's very restrictive, and many people won't accept this very low-fat way of eating. But the message is clear. All the experts agree on the need for a lower fat intake. They just can't agree on how low.

Let's look at the common high-fat foods we consume and see where we should make some adjustments.

MEAT, POULTRY, AND FISH

All animal products contain cholesterol and fat. Most red meats are especially high in saturated fats. Consumption of red meats, such as beef, pork, and lamb, should be severely limited. When eating red meats it is best to choose the very lean cuts and to have small portions. Contrary to popular opinion, cholesterol is not found just in the fat portion of the animal products. It is distributed equally throughout the lean tissue as well. Trimming the fat off meat does reduce the fat and eliminates some part of the cholesterol, but the lean meat still contains cholesterol. Substituting fish, chicken, and turkey for meat lowers cholesterol consumption somewhat. However, their big advantages are that they are lower in total fat and have a higher ratio of polyunsaturated to saturated fat. Of the fish, white fish, such as halibut, snapper, and sole, are good choices. Shellfish are good alternatives with the exception of lobster and shrimp, which are higher in cholesterol than fish. In chicken and turkey, only the white meat is lower in saturated fat and cholesterol (skin all poultry). Dark meat from poultry has about the same fat and cholesterol content as red meat.

FAST FOODS

Unfortunately, more people are turning to fast foods for reasons of convenience and economy. Most of us make poor selections. Fried chicken and fish sticks are no substitute for broiled chicken and fish. They are deep-fried in oil, which only adds more fat and calories to your diet. The oils most commonly used are palm or coconut oils, which are highly saturated. Shakes, hamburgers, and fries are also too high in fat, and, to make matters worse, they are often eaten together. Athletes especially abuse this practice by eating excessive amounts of these high-fat foods in one sitting.

EGGS

Eggs are an excellent food except for their extremely high cholesterol level. A medium-sized egg contains 250 milligrams of cholesterol. To adhere to a daily intake of 300 milligrams or less would require omitting all other animal products if just one egg was consumed. The cholesterol is found in the yolk only, so egg whites can be freely eaten. Americans have developed a strong and unhealthful habit of eating bacon and eggs for breakfast. Substituting oatmeal and other cereals and gradually cutting down on eggs will promote better health.

Some studies have shown that the lecithin in eggs prevents the serum cholesterol in the blood from rising, while others have shown that as many as two eggs a day did not raise the serum cholesterol level. Critics of these studies point out that these studies were not controlled and that the subjects' serum cholesterol was high to begin with. Dr. Julian Whitaker, director of the National Heart and Diabetes Institute, Huntington Beach, California, points out that the average cholesterol intake of Americans, which is 600 milligrams a day, is the saturation point. More cholesterol does not raise cholesterol levels! This would account for the fact that no increase in serum cholesterol is observed in subjects on an already high-cholesterol diet.

The most prudent action would be to follow the advice of the majority. The American Heart Association recommends no more than three egg yolks a week (remember, only the yolk contains cholesterol). This should include all foods made with eggs, as well.

DAIRY PRODUCTS

Dairy products are derived from animal sources, so they are high in saturated fats and cholesterol. It is best to eat the nonfat and low-fat dairy products.

The term "low-fat" is sometimes deceptive. What we see isn't always what we get! About 47% of the calories of whole milk are in the form of fat. So-called "low-fat" milk has only about 17% less fat, coming in at 30% total fat calories. Nonfat or skim milk has less than 1% total fat calories and is the best choice. Reducing the amount of all dairy products and substituting the very low fat products made with skim milk is an essential part of a healthy diet.

OILS AND FATS

Fats such as lard, bacon grease, and butter, which are highly saturated and high in cholesterol, can easily be reduced or eliminated in the preparation of many dishes. Using nonstick pans, quick frying in an oriental wok, and substituting defatted chicken broth for oils are a few ways to cook without fat. The use of large amounts of butter on bread, pancakes, and baked potatoes is a learned behavior, easily overcome.

Polyunsaturated vegetable oils are very low in saturated fat and have the added advantage of being cholesterol-free. They do, however, contain as many calories as butter, lard, and all other fats, and contribute significantly to total fat intake. Margarines aren't recommended because of the hydrogenation and additive content. They are really just a highly processed fat. Those who feel they must use butter should choose small amounts of natural unsalted butter. If the rest of the diet is low in cholesterol and saturated fat, this small amount shouldn't be detrimental. When buying vegetable oils choose small quantities of the "cold-pressed" oils, which must be kept refrigerated to prevent spoiling, sold at health-food stores. Most of the commercial oils are highly processed and may be lower in vitamin E.

ADDED FATS

Added fats are found in many processed foods, usually in the form of hydrogenated vegetable oils. Reading the labels shows which foods to eliminate. Most processed products containing fat are loaded with saturated fat or hydrogenated vegetable oils. Gravies, sauces, mayonnaise, and salad dressings, are all examples of products that are close to 100% pure fat. Baked goods like doughnuts, pies, cakes, breads, rolls, and biscuits are usually about 50% fat. Look for baked goods made with limited amounts of nonhydrogenated oils and those that are low in fat.

VEGETABLE OILS TO ELIMINATE

Coconut oil and palm oil are not polyunsaturated like other vegetable oils. They are extremely low in linoleic acid, the essential fatty acid required by the body, and they contribute saturated fat to the diet just as animal fats do. Unfortunately, these two fats are the ones most commonly used in processed foods and are the common choice of fast food companies for frying french fries, chicken, and fish. It is best to avoid all products that list either of these two oils on the label. Many labels say "vegetable oil (one of the following: coconut, corn, safflower)." It is safe to assume that coconut oil has been used. If the manufacturers had used a more expensive polyunsaturated oil like safflower, they certainly would have said so.

NUTS AND SEEDS

Even though nuts and seeds are highly nutritious and contain polyunsaturated oil, their consumption should be limited because they are extremely high in fat and calories. Vegetarians will sometimes eat a variety of nuts and seeds, but we must remember that true vegetarians, who eat no meat or dairy products, actually consume a low-fat diet (unless they add a lot of vegetable oils). They can tolerate the extra fat in nuts. When humans roamed the countryside, living off the land, they found and consumed very few nuts. Those they did find had to be shelled by hand. They didn't have the convenience of going to the supermarket and buying a jar of shelled nuts, so they ate very few nuts compared to what some of us consume today. An 8-ounce jar of cashew nuts contains close to 1,200 calories, 900 of which are pure fat! It doesn't look like much when held in the hand, but any avid football fan can eat that whole jar before half time! Two high-fat foods to limit are avocadoes and olives. They're both great foods, but unfortunately they contain 90% of their calories as fat.

Questions and Answers

Q: *I read recently that a report from the National Academy of Science recommended no reduction in fats and cholesterol in the diet of healthy Americans.*

A: That position was very heavily attacked by nutritional researchers, heart specialists, and governmental health agencies. It's ridiculous to recommend no change in the American diet when so much evidence exists that links vascular disease to our high-fat and high-cholesterol diet. Government officials pointed out that the report was financed by food companies and that many of the board members had affiliations with food companies and food lobbies. Keep in mind that if we wait for direct evidence of the link between fats and heart disease, it may be too late for many of us. Prudent dietary changes that improve your overall health are more worthwhile.

Q: *I thought fat had more energy than protein and carbohydrates.*
A: The word "energy" confuses most people when used in this respect. What we mean is that it has more *calories*. Calories are referred to as energy. Fat has nine calories in a gram, whereas protein and carbohydrates each have four calories per gram. Therefore, fat yields more energy. Unfortunately, you can't utilize dietary fat as a fuel as well as you can carbohydrates. Fats require more oxygen to burn than carbohydrates, so as a fuel their efficiency is less than that of carbohydrates, which are our most efficient energy fuel. At low levels of energy expenditure fats, carbohydrates, and a minimal amount of proteins are used as energy.

Q: *I was told that polyunsaturated oil prevents heart disease. Is that true?*
A: That was an oversimplification promoted mostly by margarine and oil distributors. At one time it was suggested that we increase our polyunsaturated oil intake to lower cholesterol. This is not particularly desirable in view of the evidence relating polyunsaturated fats to cancer. Everyone liked the idea, though—eat all the fat and sugar you want and just drop a tablespoon of oil or margarine in your mouth and you're saved! These oils may be better for you than animal fat, but lowering total fat intake is still the best advice.

Q: *I thought peanut butter was a good source of protein. Isn't it a good substitute for fatty meat?*

A: Peanut butter is 71% fat, 17% protein, and 12% carbohydrate. Do you still think it's a protein food? It also has 581 calories in 3½ ounces. Why not a tuna sandwich? Tuna is only 6% fat and 87% protein and has only 127 calories in 3½ ounces (water packed, no oil).

Q: *If I eliminate meat, will I lower my fat and cholesterol intake?*
A: Yes, especially if you eat a lot of meat. Thirty percent or more of the fat in the average American's diet comes from meat. But don't stop there. Evaluate all of your fat sources.

Q: *I've heard that fat and cholesterol are only problems for older people.*
A: That's when it catches up with you and causes disability and sometimes death. The high-fat, high-cholesterol diets of young people predispose them to atherosclerosis in later life. High levels of both cholesterol and triglycerides have been found in elementary school children who eat the typical American diet. Autopsies done on soldiers who died in the Korean War showed that they had a considerable amount of occlusion in their artery lining, from slight thickening to complete closures coronary arteries. As many as 77% showed a narrowing of the (blockage). This would not be surprising if it were found in older Americans, but in this case it involved soldiers with an average age of twenty-two years! This same study, with similar results, was duplicated in Vietnam. Dr. Ernest Wynder, of the American Health Foundation, reported on a study of 17,000 children (ages ten to fourteen) in fifteen counties. Even at this early age high blood-cholesterol level predicts the later risk of heart disease.

Q: *Can't some people escape atherosclerosis even though they eat a high-fat diet?*
A: I'm sure they can, but we can't determine who those persons might be. It would be foolish to assume you won't get atherosclerosis and, therefore, to keep eating a high-fat and high-cholesterol diet. Dr. William Castelli, director of Framingham Heart Study, reminds us that although 50% of Americans die from atherosclerotic lesions in their blood vessels, 70% of Americans die *with* these lesions, even though they may die of other causes.

Q: *I'm afraid that if I don't eat any fat I'll become malnourished. Don't we need fat in our diet?*
A: Yes, we need fat in our diet, but not very much. The body can synthesize all of the fats it needs from carbohydrate and protein except for linoleic acid, which is essential. Linoleic acid is found in polyunsaturated oils as well as in whole grains, vegetables, and fruits. Nathan Pritikin, of the Pritikin Longevity Center in Santa Monica, California, suggests that we need no more than 1/10 ounce of linoleic acid daily, an amount found in one ounce of oatmeal. If that amount seems like too little, remember that all foods have some fat. It is unlikely that you could reduce your dietary fat to much lower than 10% of your total calories, even if you eliminated all obvious fat from your diet. As hard as you try, it will be difficult to reach that low level. There has never been a fat deficiency in human beings. That's why there is no recommendation for the amount you need in your diet.

Q: *I have friends who jog every day. They say it protects them from heart disease, so they don't worry about how much fat they eat.*
A: That's a misconception many athletes, as well as physical fitness buffs, have. Exercise plays a major role in the prevention of heart disease, but there is a point of diminishing returns. First, you probably don't burn cholesterol like you do fats. Exercise does lower fat and cholesterol levels but it probably can't counteract the effect of a high-fat and high-cholesterol diet by itself. People who exercise and don't monitor their fat intake would be well advised to have a blood test to establish their blood levels of cholesterol and triglycerides. If your cholesterol is not below 200 milligrams per 100 milliliters of blood, then I suggest you lower your fat intake. We are all biologically different, so evaluation is important in determining if we are making the life-style changes that best suit us as individuals. A healthy approach is to involve yourself in a vigorous aerobic fitness program *and* to limit your fat intake.

Q: *I've been told that our body makes cholesterol and that if we didn't have cholesterol in our diet our body would just make more.*

A: It's true that the body manufactures cholesterol. The mistake we make is adding still more from our diet. Some nutritionists have said that you can't reduce the cholesterol level through your diet. Recent research shows that you can. By greatly reducing the fat and cholesterol in the diet you can lower your cholesterol level significantly. Books that imply that the cholesterol level is not significantly reduced by diet refer to diets that don't lower the total fat and cholesterol enough. Nathan Pritikin, Director of the Pritikin Longevity Center, has had very good results in lowering the blood serum cholesterol level of his patients with a fat intake of 10% of total calories.

Q: *What is a good cholesterol reading? Mine is 230 mg. and my doctor says that's average.*
A: The problem is one of interpretation. According to Dr. William Castelli, scientific director of the Framingham Study, the average American cholesterol level is 210–230 mg. He considers this a dangerously high level. As I mentioned in the text, most doctors concerned with prevention of heart disease prefer a cholesterol level under 200 mg. Dr. Castelli considers a cholesterol level of 150–160 mg. a much safer level but probably only obtainable in a vegetarian diet.

Q: *If I have atherosclerosis can it be reversed through diet adjustment?*
A: Nathan Pritikin has held that belief for a long time. He has advocated a diet with less than 10% fat content and exercise. His theory seems to have gained support from a recent research done by Dr. Dean Ornish of Baylor University and reported in the *Journal of the American Medical Association.* Dr. Ornish demonstrated objective as well as subjective benefits from a low-fat (total vegetarian except for non-fat yogurt) diet and stretching exercises along with stress reduction techniques. Eating fewer animal products seems to be a prudent diet approach for both prevention and correction of heart disease.

Q: *I was told that cholesterol was an essential part of every cell in the body. Is that true?*

A: Yes. It is essential to every cell; that's why the body manufactures it from the foods we eat! It's the *excess* we get through our diet that we should control. If you didn't consume any cholesterol, your body would make all that is required for good health.

Q: *Aren't we eliminating very nutritious foods when we don't eat meat, eggs, ice cream, cheese, butter, etc.?*
A: To some degree, yes. But there are many other foods just as nutritious. Americans are very spoiled when it comes to what they eat. Half of the world's population consumes diets with few or no animal products. Strict vegetarians experience excellent health without them. It's doubtful that you were meant to eat a breakfast of two eggs, four strips of bacon, hash browns, and pancakes everyday!

Q: *I've heard that Eskimos eat a high-fat diet and have a low incidence of heart disease. Is that true?*
A: No. the Eskimo diet is estimated to be about 23% fat. That's considerably less than our average of 42%. Much of the Eskimo diet is also high in unsaturated fat (from fish). Additionally, the incidence of breast cancer in Eskimos is high.

Q: *Should I use polyunsaturated oils for frying?*
A: No. Vegetable oils do not handle high heat very well, and frying requires too much heat. Fried oils become rancid and are very unhealthy. You should limit your intake of fried foods. If you must fry, use butter. But be aware of the amount of fat and cholesterol this adds to your total fat intake.

Q: *What's all this HDL business? I read in the newspaper that if you had a high HDL blood reading you were immune to heart disease.*
A: Confusion is great, isn't it? I'm sure the experts throw up their hands in despair when they read articles like that. Let's see if we can shed some light on the issue.

Cholesterol is carried in the blood by two major proteins: HDL (High Density Lipoprotein) and LDL (Low Density Lipoprotein). LDL is involved with carrying cholesterol to and depositing it in the tissue. HDL is involved with removing cholesterol from sites where it is in excess and carrying it to the liver for disposal. It is true that a high HDL level is associated with less coronary disease, but it is also true that a low LDL level is just as important. The ratio of the two is the most important factor. Dr. H. Bryan Brewer, Jr., M.D. of the National Heart, Lung, and Blood Institute, points out that a favorable blood test would show a low level of LDL and a high level of HDL. A low-fat diet seems to lower the LDL, which causes the damage, and vigorous exercise seems to raise the HDL, which guards against disease. Dr. Peter D. Wood of Stanford found that men between thirty-five and fifty-nine years of age who run at least fifteen miles a week had significantly higher HDL levels. It is important to note that their total cholesterol was 200 milligrams. Women seem to have a high HDL level until menopause; then it drops. This may account for some of the immunity that young women seem to have from heart disease. The best advice is to involve yourself in vigorous aerobic exercises to raise the HDL and to control your fat intake to lower the LDL and total cholesterol. Having a high HDL level is not very important if total cholesterol and LDL are not considered. An HDL of 50 and a LDL of 200 would give you a total cholesterol of 250 milligrams. Even with the high HDL, few doctors would consider that a healthy level.

Q: *What blood tests are most important with regard to my risk of heart disease?*
A: It depends on the approach of your doctor, but most specialists with an interest in prevention would look for the following:

1. Total Cholesterol: Under 200 mg.
2. HDL Cholesterol: 35–65 mg.
3. LDL Cholesterol: 170 mg. or less
4. Ratio LDL/HDL: Low
5. Ratio Cholesterol/HDL: 4.5:1 or less
6. Triglycerides: Under 100 mg.

If you have not had these blood tests, it would be a wise preventive measure to have them. A doctor knowledgeable in their significance will be able to interpret your tests and explain them to you.

Q: *What are triglycerides?*
A: Most of the fats in your food and body are called the triglycerides. They are made of glycerol attached to three fatty acids. High levels are associated with a higher incidence of heart disease. It seems that as triglyceride levels go up our serum level of low density lipoproteins goes up also. This would increase our ratio of LDL to HDL, which is more indicative of heart disease. You can lower your triglyceride level by losing weight, exercising, eating less fat, and avoiding sugar which, in excess, is converted to triglyceride.

Q: *I thought linolenic fatty acid and linoleic acid were essential fats in our diet.*
A: That's true. So is arachidonic fatty acid. Both can be manufactured by the body from linoleic acid.

Q: *I'm confused about the difference between serum cholesterol and dietary cholesterol.*
A: Serum cholesterol is a blood reading you get when you take a blood test. This reading should be low, about 200 milligrams per 100 milliliters. The amount of total fat, saturated fat, and cholesterol you eat can affect this level. Dietary cholesterol is the amount you eat in milligrams. The average American consumes 600 milligrams a day and should lower this intake to 300 milligrams or less. Simply eating fewer animal products will reduce your dietary intake of cholesterol.

3

PROTEIN:
LESS IS BETTER

Americans seem to be obsessed with the idea that protein is the most important nutrient—the more the better! To most people, protein means animal products like meat, fish, eggs, milk, and cheese. Few think that beans, whole grains, fruits, and vegetables also contain protein. This misunderstanding has been perpetuated by the meat, egg, and dairy industries, because the last thing they want us to do is eat fewer of their profitable products.

As a society, Americans not only eat too much protein but eat too much of the wrong kind. As we will see, this habit not only affects our health, but accounts for considerable waste of our food dollar.

What is Protein?

Protein's function has contributed to the myth that more is better. It is essential for the growth and maintenance of new tissue, such as muscle, hair, nails, and blood cells. It is also important in enzyme and hormone production and the formation of antibodies, and it acts as a buffer in the acid-base balance of the body.

A less important function is its ability to serve as an alternate energy source. This ability has become the rationale for high-protein weight-loss diets, high-energy diets, and a host of other unsound diet practices. These half-truth diets are often unhealthful, but they do make money for the people who promote them to a gullible public.

Protein contains the "building blocks" called amino acids. A chain may be composed of as many as 300 amino acids units. When protein is eaten, the body breaks down the amino acids into new forms that can be used for growth and maintenance functions.

Nature gave our bodies the ability to synthesize most of the amino acids—as long as we eat the essential ones. There are eight essential amino acids. If we consume these, the body can synthesize the additional amino acids required for health.

Complete or Incomplete: Which is Best?

The terms "complete" and "incomplete" have caused more confusion than any others of protein study. They imply that complete proteins are "good" and incomplete are "bad." That is not the case.

Foods containing protein that can be both digested and utilized by the body receive a "Net Protein Utilization" rating. Eggs, the reference point against which all other protein foods are measured, have an NPU of 95. Animal products such as eggs, meats, and poultry are good examples of "complete proteins" because they contain all the eight essential amino acids in adequate amounts.

Incomplete proteins are usually deficient in one or more of the essential amino acids. Plant foods such as grains, nuts, peas, rice, and beans fall into this category. For years people have believed that we must eat complete proteins (meat, fish, or fowl), because they have the essential amino acids our bodies require, or we will suffer protein deficiency. We often hear, "Eat all your meat if you want big muscles," or "Drink four glasses of milk a day," or "Eggs are perfect food, eat all you want." Who promoted these ideas? Obviously they are untrue, since over half the world's population receives adequate protein on a diet totally free of animal products.

Combining Foods for Protein

In the United States we are so accustomed to eating high on the food chain—that is, eating animal products high in protein—that we forget that most of the world survives on plant protein. The important point to remember is that plants contain the same essential amino acids that animal foods do.

Plant foods can be just as complete in amino acids as animal products if they are eaten in the correct combination. For example, grains and legumes, which are low in certain amino acids, become complete when eaten together. Rice is deficient in the amino acid lysine but high in methionine, while beans are high in the amino acids lysine and tryptophan but low in methionine. Eaten alone, they are incomplete. Eaten together, however, they have as many amino acids as a steak! Other excellent common combinations might be rice and wheat or legumes and corn. The legumes (beans, peas, etc.) are an excellent plant food to include in the diet to ensure an adequate protein intake.

Our Protein Requirements

The recommended daily allowance of protein is very generous. For example, the recommendation for men is 56 grams a day, while for women it is 44 grams. Children, infants, pregnant women, and nursing mothers require more protein to accommodate for growth and maintenance. The R.D.A. (Recommended Dietary Allowance) for protein is established by the National Academy of Science on the basis of scientific studies that determine our needs according to body weight. An adult requires 0.36 grams of protein per pound of body weight. Be sure that you use your "ideal body weight," since your fat weight is not as significant as your lean weight in determining protein needs. Infants require about 1 gram per pound of body weight, while the requirements for growing children range from 0.81 to 0.39 gram, decreasing as they get older. Pregnant and nursing women should receive about 0.62 gram of protein per pound of body weight.

EXAMPLES

150 pound male: $150 \times 0.36 = 52.5$ grams
110 pound female: $110 \times 0.36 = 39.6$ grams

Including Protein in Your Diet

An interesting point, which is seldom clarified, is that only 20% of our protein requirement must come from essential amino acids. Essential amino acids are much better utilized when combined with a mixed diet of plant food that is sufficient in total calories.

Even a vegetarian will easily get enough protein as long as he or she understands how to combine foods (for example, beans and rice). Nonvegetarians should substantially reduce consumption of animal protein. Many Americans consume in excess of 100 grams of animal protein a day. If 20% of our protein requirement was derived from animal products (complete protein) we would be assured of receiving sufficient quantities of the eight essential amino acids. The remainder of our daily requirement should come from plant foods (legumes, grains, vegetables, and fruit).

The following chart provides a perspective on the amount of protein found in animal sources:

PROTEIN IN ANIMAL PRODUCTS

	Amount	Protein
Meat (steak, pork, lamb)	3 ounces	22 grams
Fish	3 ounces	22 grams

PROTEIN IN ANIMAL PRODUCTS (continued)

	Amount	Protein
Poultry	3 ounces	22 grams
Egg	One	6 grams
Milk	1 cup	9 grams
Cheese	1 ounce	7 grams
Cottage Cheese	1 cup	33 grams

The point I want to make is that our protein needs can be met without consuming large amounts of animal protein. Let's take our average adult male who requires fifty-six grams of protein a day. If he eats 20% of his requirement from animal foods he would only need 11.2 grams. That's about two ounces of meat a day. If the rest of his daily food intake was composed of mixed plant foods such as beans, grain, fruits, and vegetables, which also supply protein, then his diet would more than likely be adequate in protein. Let's look at an example of how easy it would be to get 56 grams of protein:

Bread (2 slices)	4 grams
Potato (7 ounces)	4 grams
Kidney Beans (1/2 cup)	7 grams
Oatmeal (1 cup)	5 grams
Skim Milk (1 cup)	9 grams
Spaghetti (1 cup)	7 grams
Chicken (3 ounces)	22 grams
	58 grams

How valid is the R.D.A. for protein? The R.D.A., which is determined by The National Academy of Sciences, is actually a high figure. The minimum requirement is about 30% less. Your goal should not be to see how low you can get but, rather, to realize how little you really need. The requirement already has an allowance built in for additional requirements that may arise.

The Benefits
of Eating Plant Protein

Most nutritionists and doctors recommend that we eat less animal protein and shift our diet toward mixed plants for the majority of our food.

Let's look at some of the advantages:

1. Plant foods are lower in saturated fat.
2. Plants do not contain cholesterol.
3. Plants are high in essential fiber.
4. Plants can be complete in protein when combined with other plant foods (for example, grains with legumes).
5. Most plant foods are low in calories.
6. Plant foods are high in complex carbohydrates (animal tissue does not contain carbohydrates).

Problems with Too Much Protein

The myths about the magical qualities of proteins have been perpetuated for generations. It is time we take a look at the cold hard facts about overconsumption of protein, especially in the form of animal products.

Many protein foods are among the most expensive foods, so overconsumption is a waste of money. Additionally, too much of this type of food may contribute to kidney problems, gout, mineral deficiency, and all of the problems associated with high fat and cholesterol intake.

ENERGY AND PROTEIN

Complex carbohydrates, not protein, are the best energy source. It is true that when carbohydrates are not available to our cells the body converts protein to glucose, which can then be used for our energy needs. This happens if we fast or starve ourselves. But that's like lighting a fire with dollars bills rather than paper! We should eat a reasonable amount of protein, leaving it to serve its main purpose of growth and maintenance, eating the less costly complex carbohydrates for energy.

FAT AND CHOLESTEROL

Animal products are our major source of saturated fat and cholesterol. As previously discussed, these are two of the major dietary risk factors associated with atherosclerosis. Reducing our intake of animal products will result in a corresponding decrease in saturated fat and cholesterol.

KIDNEYS

Excess protein intake puts an overload on the kidneys as they attempt to eliminate nitrogen in the form of urea. Those with existing kidney problems and older people whose kidney function is less than optimal should avoid excessive intake of protein. Avoid especially organ meats and high-protein diets, with their associated high fat content; they elevate the uric acid level and can cause gout in susceptible individuals.

CANCER

Scientific evidence has begun to indicate that high-protein diets may be associated with certain cancers. Some authorities link cancer more to the fat associated with meat, while still others blame the use of hormones and antibiotics used in raising livestock. Diethylstilbestrol (DES), a known carcinogen, is used in commercial beef. The Federal Food and Drug Administration says that only small amounts of the chemical are allowed, but that policing beef products is difficult. "Faith" that the beef producers will do the right thing is the major control. As recently as September of 1980 the FDA found 55 distributors and 424 cattle feeders using DES. Given the distribution, it is probable that every consumer of beef products was affected.

Cancer of the colon, diverticulitis, and other diseases of the intestine have been associated with a diet high in meat and fat and low in fiber.

There is still widespread debate in the scientific community over the exact causes of these diseases. Some scientists maintain that the meat is the culprit, while others blame lack of fiber. Until the evidence is more conclusive, the prudent and healthy approach to the problem is to lower meat consumption and increase the amount of fiber in the diet.

OSTEOPOROSIS

Osteoporosis is a condition in which bone density is reduced due to calcium depletion. This condition makes the bones weak, which makes them more susceptible to fracture. Adequate calcium intake and exercise are two main factors in the possible prevention of osteoporosis, but there is a strong indication that too much protein reduces calcium absorption and increases calcium loss.

OBESITY AND OVERWEIGHT

Contrary to popular opinion, overconsumption of high-fat animal protein is responsible for most of the obesity and overweight in this country. Protein actually has the same amount of calories as carbohydrates, but in animal products it is combined with fats which increase total calories. While dining out it is not uncommon to see people eat a 12-ounce top sirloin steak and avoid bread and potatoes because they are considered fattening foods. Actually, a baked potato contains only 145 calories and bread only about 75 calories per slice. The 12-ounce steak has about 1,200 calories! It would be much better to choose smaller portions of low-fat animal products and eat more plant foods that are low-fat to control calorie intake.

The Effect of Protein
on Athletic Performance

Some American athletes eat well over 250 grams a day of high-quality protein in the form of eggs, meat, fish, milk, and cheese in the belief that it will enhance performance and build strong muscles. This infatuation with protein not only fails to build muscles and enhance performance but actually can do considerable harm. Protein does so many useful things like replacing tissue and building blood cells, hormones, and enzymes that it's hard to believe that more is not better.

Protein Requirements
of Athletes

An almost endless number of laboratory studies, as well as population studies, emphasize the minimal protein requirements of humans. While many athletes gorge themselves with as much as 200 to 300 grams of protein a day, Indians in the Andes Highlands ride bicycles 150 miles at 24 miles per hour and the Tarahumara Indians run 90 miles at 7 miles per hour on a protein intake well below 50 grams! The Equatorial Highlanders of New Guinea are exceptionally healthy and do strenuous physical work on a protein intake of 15 to 20 grams a day. Athletes have been conned into believing that they need more protein than sedentary people. This idea has spread by association. Body builders still cling to the high-protein philosophy and encourage young athletes to increase their intake with protein supplements. The logic is there! When a young athlete hears a successful athlete with bulging muscles say that protein is the reason for success it's hard to dispute the fact. Actually, it's hard work that stimulates muscle growth. Protein plays a much less significant role. Trained athletes assimilate protein more efficiently than inactive people and may even require less protein! The studies that suggest any increased need for protein are talking about an increased need in "excess of the R.D.A." and not an increase in what you may now be eating. For the sake of argument, let's assume that your R.D.A. is 56 grams of protein a day. If you buy the argument that you need more you may want to increase your intake by 10%; that's 5.6 grams a day for a total of 61.6 grams. *No studies have ever suggested that you should double your R.D.A.!* Since the R.D.A. already has a 30% allowance built in it seems pointless to go much higher. You can be assured that as soon as I see proof that a considerable increase in dietary protein improves performance, I'll be the first to support it. Don't hold your breath waiting, though.

Protein for Energy

If a book says that protein is needed for energy, throw it away. If someone lectures on the value of protein as an energy source, walk away. These people are uninformed "experts." Protein's main function is to replace body tissue, which is constantly being broken down. If the diet is sufficient to meet this need, then any excess is converted to fat and stored as body fat. Some protein (about 10%) is used for energy, but this is not significant compared to the contribution carbohydrates make to our energy needs. The body always considers its energy needs first. During a total fast the body starts breaking down muscle tissue (protein) to meet its energy needs. However, if we eat a high-carbohydrate diet, our need for protein actually goes down. Because the carbohydrates are properly meeting our energy needs, the protein is "spared" to go about its job of replacing muscle tissue, hormones, enzymes, etc. It's important that athletes realize how important carbohydrates are to energy. Eating a high-protein diet from animal products that are also high in fat can reduce your energy level considerably because it reduces your carbohydrate intake. To assume that protein provides energy as effectively as carbohydrates is much like saying that pushing a car is as efficient as running it on gas!

Protein for Building Muscles

Some ill-informed trainers and coaches are still recommending high-protein diets and protein supplements to athletes who train with weights. Let's see if we can shed some light on how a muscle grows and what relationship protein has to that growth.

It is true that as muscle size increases the need for protein increases. The point everyone overlooks is that a muscle grows in size very gradually; therefore, the increased need for protein is gradual. If an exercise increased caloric needs from 1,500 calories to 2,500 calories a day, those doing it would not think they were better off to eat 4,000 calories! That would meet their energy needs all right, but the excess calories would be converted to fat. The same is true with protein. Any excess just turns to fat.

The first and most important step in muscle growth is *stimulation.* Just about any stress exercise will provide this stimulation, but high-intensity exercises, such as weight training, are most effective. Given proper stimulation, the muscle will grow even on a low-protein vegetarian diet. The daily need for extra protein is infinitely small. Let's assume that under normal conditions the protein requirement is 50 grams a day. Someone who decides to lift weights on a regular basis in an effort to "stimulate" more muscle growth will need more protein. A pound of muscle is about 20% (or 100 grams) protein. If our weight lifter increases his or her muscle mass by one pound every ten days (a great amount!), how much additional protein will he or she need on a daily basis? The answer: only 10 grams per day (100 grams of protein divided by 10 days). This small daily need is easily met in any reasonable diet. How soon we forget all the successful football players, weight lifters, and body builders who are vegetarians. They eat no meat, limited dairy products, and no protein supplements, and yet they develop beautifully formed muscles.

Protein Supplements

Makers of protein supplements say that athletes should take them for the following reasons:

1. They can increase the protein content of the normal diet.
2. They offer a high-quality protein that can be utilized by the body.
3. They meet the additional protein requirements of athletes seeking to build muscle mass.
4. They meet the energy needs of athletic performance.

The protein need of athletes is so easily met from the normal diet that the small contribution a supplement makes is insignificant. A tablespoon of protein powder or a handful of protein pills yields about 15 grams of protein. Four ounces of meat, fish, etc. yields 28 grams of protein. The value of eating the protein in the form of food is the natural balance of other nutrients such as vitamins and minerals that are present in the food but not in the concentrated supplement. The implication that protein supplements supply a higher quality, more utilizable protein is absurd! The supplements are derived from food, usually in the form of egg albumen, and milk. Surely eating the egg or drinking the milk provides the highest quality protein. The suggestion that we need to eat large amounts of animal protein is not supported by any scientific proof. Vegetable protein can adequately meet the needs of athletes, especially in the presence of *small* amounts of low-fat animal protein. We have already discussed the relationship of energy and muscle tissue replacement. Additional protein plays a minimal role in muscle growth and has a negative affect on energy.

For best results, the athlete should eat a diet low in protein and high in complex carbohydrates. The protein needs of athletes can range from 10% of their total calories in endurance events to 15% in strength events. Eating less animal protein by substituting plant protein and avoiding protein supplementation will produce the best results. For the development of muscle mass and strength, hard training on resistive weights (stimulus) should be emphasized, while energy and protein needs are met through a balanced diet. Excessive dietary protein does not stimulate muscle development. The excess is either stored as fat or, when carbohydrates are limited, used for energy, not an efficient process to obtain optimum performance.

Questions and Answers

Q: *Isn't protein a good source or energy? I heard you can convert over 50% of your protein intake to energy.*
A: No, to the first part. Protein is a very poor energy souce. Carbohydrate is the cleanest and best fuel the body can use. If your body is lacking in carbohydrates, it will convert protein to carbohydrate for energy, but complex carbohydrates from plant foods are a more efficient and economical way to provide energy. Let protein do what it does best: develop growth and maintenance of tissue.

Q: *I work as a laborer all day and jog 10 miles a day. Don't I need more protein?*
A: No. You may even need less! If you get enough calories for your energy needs, your protein need goes down. High protein intake can cause dehydration, which can affect your athletic performance.

Q: *I thought that the major world hunger problem was a protein deficiency.*
A: No. The problem is not enough calories and not enough variety of plant food. Eating more protein without enough calories to meet the body's energy needs will not solve the problem. Protein deficiency has never been found in adults in the United States.

Q: *What do you mean when you say a person needs less protein when they get enough calories in their diet?*
A: Given enough calories in the form of carbohydrates and fats, the body does not have to break down protein for energy. Therefore, your protein is "spared" and used for its most important function, growth and repair.

Q: *What would happen if I ate a "high-protein diet" of just eggs, meat, and fish?*
A: With regard to protein specifically, your body would convert some protein to glucose to meet its energy needs. Any excess would be converted to fat and stored (resulting in weight gain).

This would be like burning one hundred-dollar bills for a fire when less expensive and better-burning fuels (carbohydrates) are available.

Q: *What happens if I eat more protein than I need?*
A: Excess protein is converted to fat and stored while the nitrogen is excreted through the kidneys as urea.

Q: *I notice I lose weight on a high-protein diet. What do you think?*
A: Yes, you do lose *weight* but not much fat! Most of the weight is in the form of water. The more protein you eat, the more water you need to eliminate the waste products of protein metabolism. The body will draw this water from its cells, causing temporary weight loss. That loss is regained when you replace the lost fluid by drinking water or eating foods high in water content.

Q: *Aren't carbohydrates more fattening than proteins?*
A: No. Actually, they yield the same amount of calories. Protein and carbohydrates yield 4 calories per gram of food. Fats yield 9 calories per gram. No food is really "fattening." If you eat more calories of *any* food, then you will gain weight.

Q: *What about liquid-protein diets?*
A: Stay away from them! You only get about 300 calories a day on this kind of diet. This causes a considerable loss of potassium, which may be the cause of the few deaths that occurred when these products first came on the market. They are a "stopgap" measure at best in the control of obesity. Some clinics and universities have recently started weight-loss programs for obese people using liquid protein. They are directed by knowledgeable medical professionals and include constant monitoring of patients' blood chemistry. Eventually they assist patients in changing to proper eating habits, which is very important. Contact your local university's medical department for the names of *reputable* programs in your area.

Q: *Won't I become deficient in vitamin B_{12} if I eat less meat?*
A: A deficiency is doubtful unless you eliminate *all* animal protein from your diet. If you are getting 20% of your protein from animal sources, you will not suffer B_{12} deficiency from a

lack in your diet. In fact, some doctors believe that the body may be able to synthesize B_{12} when animal protein is not available. There is also some B_{12} in plant food.

Q: *How do strict vegetarians, who eat no animal protein, get by?*
A: Vegetarians study plant food combinations. Once they understand the mixtures of plant foods that yield the best protein combinations, adequate nutrition becomes very easy. Most vegetarians include dairy products in their diet, which ensures sufficient protein intake.

Q: *Do you have to eat more plant protein to get your requirement?*
A: Yes, but that's no problem. Plant foods are lower in calories, so you can eat greater quantities without ill effects.

Q: *Can a high-protein diet contribute to dehydration during exercise?*
A: Yes. Excessive protein intake can contribute to dehydration by drawing water from the body tissues to dilute urea and eliminate it through the kidneys. This is hardly a desirable state for maximum performance.

Q: *But can't protein be converted to glucose and used as an energy source?*
A: Yes. If your body does not have enough carbohydrates, it converts protein (from your food or muscle tissue) to meet its energy demands. Using carbohydrates is more efficient and more economical. Using protein for fuel is like putting high-performance oil in a junk car.

Q: *If I eat a high-protein diet, won't I gain more muscle weight?*
A: No. You'll just get fatter. Muscles only get bigger if they're stimulated. It's the great miracle of adaptation. If you never lift a weight (resistance), you don't need more muscles and strength, so your body doesn't make more muscle.

Q: *Is there a time during training or competition when protein is used as a fuel?*
A: If the athlete has severely limited his carbohydrate intake, then protein may contribute to his energy needs. But this will

direct protein away from its main function of growth and maintenance.

Q: *Doesn't this signify the importance of adding protein to the diet?*
A: No. On the contrary, it points out the importance of eating a varied high-carbohydrate diet to "spare" the protein from being broken down and used for energy. This does not mean you should go out of your way to eat a low-protein diet, but it does emphasize the importance of not eating an excessive amount at the expense of your best fuel, carbohydrate.

Q: *What affect do steroids have on muscle development?*
A: Steroids are widely used among football players, weight lifters, and some women athletes. It's still unclear if they actually cause an increase in muscle mass. The price the athlete pays for this possible increase is high. In adolescents steroids can cause stunting, while in older athletes they can cause testicular atrophy and possible sterility. Women athletes can expect coarser skin texture and increased facial hair. As one bodybuilder put it, "It's a hell of a price to pay for a handshake and a trophy."

4
CARBOHYDRATES: OUR ENERGY SOURCE

Carbohydrates are probably the most misunderstood nutrient in our diet. Many of us who have a weight problem will avoid them because they are considered to be fattening foods, while others, such as athletes, will consume great quantities to meet the energy demands of physical exercise. Both are wrong to some degree.

Carbohydrates exist in the food chain, predominantly in plant foods. Carbohydrates are also found in dairy products and, to a lesser degree, in shellfish. If our diet contained a good amount of plant carbohydrates, we would be consuming a good diet, one providing a good energy source not only for the athlete, but for the obese as well. The problem with carbohydrates is that we change them! Generally, this is called processing food. Through processing we developed refined sugars, such as table sugar (sucrose), and refined starches, such as cookies, cakes, instant potatoes, breakfast cereals, and a host of other products. This means we have two general types of carbohydrates. Those from plant sources, in their least processed state, are complex carbohydrates, and those which are derivatives of the original carbohydrates are refined carbohydrates. For example, table sugar is processed from beets or cane sugar to give us sucrose.

This enables us to add sugar to many products and thereby increases our intake of sugar considerably. As we shall see, this "adjustment" of how we derive our carbohydrates has several undesirable effects on our health and performance.

Our Need for Sugar

We all need sugar. What we don't need is excessive amounts of it. Natural food in its whole state will supply your body with all the energy it demands, even for marathons and triathlons. In 1976 we consumed in excess of 125 pounds of refined and processed sugar per person. If that does not seem high, consider that in 1875 our average consumption was only 40 pounds per person. On the average, each of us consumes 18% of our total calories as refined and processed sugar. It is suggested that we reduce that amount to 10% or less of our total calories. Keep in mind, you could go without all refined and processed sugars. Your body will get along just fine on nature's sugar found in complex carbohydrates. Save the refined sugar for infrequent sweet treats. Since we're eating so much refined food, it's easy to understand why our intake of nutritious complex carbohydrates is so low. We each consume only about 28% of our total calories in this form. We should increase that to at least 48%. For those involved in physical performance, the intake of complex carbohydrates and naturally occurring sugars can go as high as 80%.

Different Kinds of Sugar

SIMPLE CARBOHYDRATES

All carbohydrates contain sugar. Those of nutritional significance are the "simple sugars," called monosaccharides. The main monosaccharides are fructose, glucose, and galactose. These monosaccharides combine to make the disaccharides. Glucose and fructose form sucrose; glucose and galactose form lactose, glucose and glucose form maltose. Sucrose is found in honey, fruits, and more commonly as table sugar, a concentrated form of sugar extracted from sugar beets and sugar cane. Lactose is milk sugar, while maltose is malt sugar.

COMPLEX CARBOHYDRATES

Starches make up the majority of our dietary complex carbohydrates. They are referred to as polysaccharides, which are branched chains of many glucose molecules. Starches are the plants' stores of energy. Grains, beans, corn, and potatoes are examples of starch foods. They are excellent sources of energy.

REFINED SUGARS

The disaccharide sucrose is the most widely used refined sugar. Unlike the sugars found in fruits, grains, and vegetables, refined sugars supply only energy, since they are extracted from the plants without the benefit of vitamins, minerals, and fiber. Because they are in highly concentrated form, it is quite easy for us to consume too much sugar. Other highly concentrated sugars that fit in this category are fructose, glucose, dextrose, corn syrup, corn sugar, honey, invert sugar, molasses, and maple sugar.

Defeating Mother Nature

Food technology has played a major role in "adjusting" complex carbohydrates to the point where they are frequently no longer a natural product. Rather than improving the food by increasing its nutritional value, food technologists have simply manipulated the food for their own profit, producing many convenience foods that are less than nutritionally adequate. The following are a few isolated examples of how food technology defeats Mother Nature.

MILLING FLOUR FROM GRAINS

Grain, a natural carbohydrate, has three main parts: the bran, which is the outside portion that contains important fiber; the endosperm, which contains starch and protein; and the germ, which is high in a variety of nutrients, especially vitamins and minerals. When grains are milled into white flour the bran and germ are removed, leaving only the endosperm, which is high in starch but low in fiber, vitamins, and minerals. This product is promoted as white flour, the base for white-flour products. "Enriched flour" isn't much better, since the processor just adds back four or five nutrients, usually thiamine (B_1), riboflavin (B_2), niacin (B_3) and iron. That may sound great, but the grain started with over twenty nutrients! (The removal of the germ and bran during the milling of white flour eliminates from 60 to 80% of the vitamins and minerals, about 26 in all.) Dr. Roger J. Williams, in his book *Nutrition and Disease,* suggests that enriched flour should be called "deficient flour." Enriched flour is found not only in white breads but in all other white-flour products such as cakes, cookies, crackers, pastries, doughnuts, biscuits, muffins, waffles, pancakes, macaroni, and noodles. These products have the added attraction of refined sugar.

A word on breakfast cereals. Most of the popular cereals on the market are a blend of enriched flours and refined sugars baked into funny little forms that kids love. Packaged foods list ingredients in descending order; the ingredients listed first are those contained in the food in the largest quantity. In the list on cereal boxes we find that some cereals have more sugar than cereal! Hard to believe, but true. What kind of doctor and dental bills must parents encounter when their child starts eating a cereal with a refined sugar content of 54%, not to mention the artificial colors, preservatives, and additives? It's best to avoid the highly processed cereals altogether. Natural cereals, such as oatmeal, and mixed grains with added sugar are good choices. Mixed grains brought in bulk are nutritious and less expensive; but beware of "granolas" with added honey, nuts, coconut, and turbino sugars. They may be higher in sugar, fat and calories than the highly processed product.

THE HIDDEN SUGAR IN PROCESSED FOODS

If we could make a generalization about the sugar content of the average American diet it would be: "The more processed foods in our diet, the more sugar we eat." This is true even when you eliminate the obvious junk such as soft drinks, candy, pastry, cakes, and pies. The amount of refined sugar used by food processors has more than doubled since 1965, until today 70% of our refined sugar consumption comes from processed foods.

Looking for something to drink? We know we should eliminate soft drinks, but what can we have? Which of the following popular drinks would have a low amount of sugar?

1. Hi "C" Orange Drink
2. Tang (orange juice substitute)
3. Kool-Aid

The answer is "none of the above." Of the total calories, Hi "C" is 87% sugar; Tang, 93% sugar, and Kool-Aid, 98% sugar. They are almost entirely refined sugar and water. A nutritious selection would be orange juice. Just an ordinary orange squeezed through a juicer will provide vitamins, minerals, and fiber, as well as natural sugar.

For another example of hidden sugar, let's consider the peach, a healthy, low-calorie carbohydrate food. The label on canned peaches in heavy syrup discloses that 61% of the calories are sugar. Water-packed peaches have no added sugar, which means that when we eat peaches in heavy syrup we get a refined sugar and three times the calories—but we don't get a single extra peach!

Refined sugar is in almost everything we can imagine. Food producers want to attract our sweet tooth to "hook" us on their products. We find sugar in the most innocent-looking foods. Things like mayonnaise, catsup, nondairy creamers, jelly, spaghetti sauces, gelatin desserts, T.V. dinners, frozen and canned foods, and packaged mixes are loaded with unneeded refined sugar. Some inconspicuous food products and their sugar contents are: Hamburger Helper, 23%; Jello, 82%; Shake-and-

Bake, 50%; Heinz Ketchup, 29%; Quaker 100% Natural Cereal, 24%; Coffee-mate Non-Dairy Creamer, 65%; General Mills Breakfast Squares, 40%.

To be healthy today requires shifting the diet away from overprocessed foods, which are high in refined sugars, and eating more plant foods—fruits, vegetables, and whole-grain products.

Digesting Carbohydrates

The sugar contained in all food is eventually released during digestion to form glucose. Stored in the liver and muscle tissues, glucose supplies a readily available fuel for our body's energy requirements.

Although the end product, glucose, is the same whether we eat simple or complex carbohydrates, there are significant reasons to choose plant foods over refined sugars. Both the manner in which the body breaks down the carbohydrate molecules and the concentration of the sugars are important factors to general health.

Complex carbohydrates contain many glucose units, sometimes several hundred, bonded together. This means that when we eat complex carbohydrates the sugar is released very slowly, supplying the body with a regulated intake of sugar. More importantly, natural foods such as fruit, whole grains, and vegetables contain fiber, which dilutes the total sugar in the food. This phenomenon is referred to as "density." For example, 100 grams of granulated table sugar (1/2 cup) yield 100 grams of sugar while one small apple (100 grams) contains only 15 grams of sugar. You would have to eat almost seven apples to ingest the same amount of sugar. Natural foods also contain the vitamins and minerals essential to sugar metabolism, while refined sugars, which do not contain vitamins and minerals, must rely on the nutrients from other foods in the diet for their metabolism.

Refined Sugar:
Why You Should Avoid It

The typical American consumes about 125 pounds of sugar a year, mostly from highly processed foods. Refined sugars are highly concentrated and contain no nutritional value—energy, yes, but they are a poor choice when other sources are available. They contribute excess calories devoid of vitamins, minerals, and fiber. The consumption of refined sugars has been associated with various negative effects, some of which are described below.

LOW BLOOD SUGAR (HYPOGLYCEMIA)

The body controls the blood sugar level with the hormone insulin, which is secreted by the pancreas. Insulin keeps the blood sugar level around 100 milligrams of glucose per 100 milliliters of blood under normal circumstances. When concentrated sugars, candy for example, are consumed, the blood is flooded with sugar. This rapid increase in the blood sugar level triggers an overreaction by the pancreas, which releases too much insulin into the bloodstream. This in turn causes a rapid drop in the blood sugar and produces the symptoms of hypoglycemia: rapid heart rate, trembling, dizziness, weakness, and hunger. To combat these symptoms most people reach for a "sugar fix," taking in more refined sugar, which starts a yo-yo cycle. Although actual hypoglycemia is very rare, it is not uncommon for people to develop the symptoms of low blood sugar when they eat excesive amounts of concentrated sugar at one time. The human body is accustomed to getting its sugar in a more diluted form, such as from fruits and vegetables. For a more normalized blood sugar this method would be the wisest choice for most of us.

DIABETES

Diabetes is the failure of the pancreas to secrete sufficient insulin to allow sugar to be taken into the cells of the body. Although development of the disease is strongly influenced by genetic tendencies and appears to be more common among obese people and those eating a high-calorie diet, many experts feel that the excessive amount of refined sugar in the diet is related to the increased incidence of the disease in this country. Many studies have shown a relationship between high incidence of diabetes and a high sugar intake. Studies have also shown that immigrants who migrate into countries with high sugar consumption have a significant increase in the incidence of diabetes, even though the disease is virtually nonexistent in their country of origin.

Individuals suffering Type I diabetes (previously referred to as juvenile onset) produce little or no insulin on their own and must take insulin to control their disease. Individuals with the more prevalent Type II diabetes (adult onset), which affects 85% of the diabetics in the United States, seem to produce insulin but are unable to utilize it normally. Their cells appear to become insulin resistant. For the Type II diabetic, a diet low in fat and refined sugar yet high in complex carbohydrates and fiber has met with considerable success in practical application. Coupled with regular exercise the Type II patient is able to reduce his or her insulin dependence, in many cases eliminating the use of medication altogether.

Dr. Jean Mayer, a leading nutritionist in the United States, points out that even though the evidence is circumstantial, the relationship between sugar and diabetes is more than an allegation. Since diabetes afflicts close to 12 million Americans and is related to atherosclerosis, stroke, heart attack, and kidney failure, any positive diet change to prevent or control the disease seems worthwhile.

HEART DISEASE

Although the major cause of heart disease is thought to be related to fats and cholesterol, there is some indication that sugar may play in important role. High sugar intake raises the level of triglycerides in the blood. Triglycerides contain fatty acids, many of which are formed when glucose is changed to fat to be stored in the body's fat cells. High triglyceride blood levels have been associated with an increased incidence of heart disease.

OBESITY AND MALNUTRITION

Refined sugar added to food products enables you to eat more calories without getting full. This increase in calories beyond your energy requirements ends up as body fat. When you eat natural carbohydrates such as fruits and vegetables you become more satisfied because natural foods are more filling. This in turn prevents you from eating an excessive number of calories.

Refined sugar is also commonly associated with fats in many processed foods. For example, one doughnut can add 125 calories to your diet: 54 calories in fat and 65 calories in refined sugar. It doesn't take long before that type of eating is compounded into a serious weight problem. We can only store a limited amount of sugar in the body; any excesses are rapidly converted to fat, which increases the amount of fat tissue carried around.

CAVITIES

Studies of populations who eat little or no refined sugar show that they are relatively free of tooth decay. When they switch to a modern diet, high in refined sugar, the incidence of tooth decay goes up. There is some controversy over how this occurs. Is it the sugar adhering to the tooth? Is it missing nutrients? The reason is not clear. However, what is clear is that people who don't eat refined sugar have a much lower incidence of cavities.

Young people who grow up on sweetened baby formulas, commercial baby food, sugar-coated cereals, soft drinks, candy, and an array of other refined foods should be ready to spend a considerable amount of their money at the dentist.

The Advantages of Complex Carbohydrates

Complex carbohydrates are found in all plant foods. They are not only the best source of energy, but probably the best foods we can eat. Starches such as grains, corn, potatoes, and fruit usually have the highest concentration of complex carbohydrates. Rather than the negative effects associated with refined sugar, complex carbohydrates have many positive advantages in a healthy diet.

1. *Slow assimilation:* Natural carbohydrates have many glucose bonds, so the blood sugar level remains stable and does not stress the pancreas for insulin. They are the best fuel for our energy needs. (Athletes take heed.) Eating refined sugar is like flooding your engine with gas. Eating complex carbohydrates is like having a carburetor to control the flow of fuel into the blood. It prevents stalling and helps your body run smoothly.

2. *High in vitamins and minerals:* All complex carbohydrates have an abundance of the natural vitamins and minerals essential to life. Special mention should be made of the B vitamins, which are essential in the metabolism of sugar and, therefore, are found in abundance in natural carbohydrates.

When one uses high amounts of refined sugar, which is devoid of B vitamins, the body must supply the vitamins from other foods. This is like "robbing Peter to pay Paul." Some nutritionists see no problem with this aspect of eating refined sugar, since they assume that the rest of the diet is high in naturally occurring vitamins. My observation of the diet patterns of students seldom substantiates that belief. It seems that students who eat the highest amount of refined sugar eat a diet very low in natural carbohydrate, with the emphasis on meat, fat, and refined products.

A diet high in complex carbohydrates will ensure proper proportions of all the minerals, especially the important trace minerals. The high-protein, high-fat diet that the western world eats is associated with calcium loss. Dr. S. Margen of the University of California at Berkeley found a calcium loss of 800% on a 90-gram (typical protein intake of the average American) protein diet. This occurred regardless of the amount of calcium supplements taken. This is a good example of nutrition. It shows that if we abuse the diet in one way (too much protein), we can't maintain the abuse and solve the problem another way (by adding calcium supplements).

3. *High in fiber:* Fiber is the cellulose or fibrous part of plants that the body cannot digest. Low-fiber diets have been associated with several diseases, especially cancer of the colon. Anyone eating a diet high in complex carbohydrates will be assured of getting an adequate amount of fiber. As an added advantage, fiber helps to slow the absorption of sugar into the system.

4. *Low in Fat:* Many of the complex carbohydrates such as fruits and vegetables are low in fat. The small amount of fat they do contain is a polyunsaturated fat, high in linoleic acid, an essential fat needed for good health. Even a strict vegetarian diet made up only of fruits, vegetables, and legumes will insure an adequate intake of fat.

5. *Cholesterol Free:* Cholesterol, which is associated with heart disease, is not found in plant foods, only in animal products.

6. *Adequate protein:* A mixed diet of complex carbohydrates will insure an adequate intake of essential amino acids. Although small amounts of animal protein are helpful, recent research indicates that animal protein is not necessary.

7. *Low in Calories:* Natural carbohydrates are low in calories. Excess calories come primarily from fat and refined sugar. Potatoes, which many people think of as fattening, contain only 93 calories per 3 1/2 ounces, yet 3 1/2 ounces of top sirloin steak with its high fat content contains 408 calories. That's over four times as many calories, yet most dieters will select steak over a potato because they think it's less fattening. The important role of complex carbohydrates in weight control will be discussed later.

Fiber: Eating More for Better Health

WHERE WE FIND FIBER

Fiber is the indigestible part of plants that supplies roughage or residue to our digestive system. It is not assimilated like other nutrients, but stays in the digestive tract, passing through the large intestine and stimulating elimination. One of the major advantages of a diet high in natural carbohydrates is their high fiber content. Only plant foods contain fiber. Animal products, sugar, white-flour products, and highly processed foods contribute little, if any, fiber to our diet. As mentioned earlier, fiber is eliminated from flour during the milling process. Thus it is eliminated from other processed products like cereals, breads, pastries, and cookies. The typical American diet rarely contains enough fiber for good health.

WHY FIBER IS IMPORTANT

Until recently, fiber was not considered important in the diet, since we don't derive any nutrients from it. However, extensive research, especially that of Dr. Dennis Burkitt, a famous English surgeon (best known for his discovery of the cancer, Burkitt's lymphoma), has generated a renewed interest in fiber's value.

Several years ago, Dr. Burkitt presented to the medical community the theory that a lack of fiber in the diet was part of the cause of several diseases, such as obesity, appendicitis, diabetes, diverticulosis, and cancer of the colon. This theory was based on research he did in Africa, where he found these diseases to be almost nonexistent. His research showed that Africans passed "bulk" through the intestinal tract faster than Englishmen. He believed that the faster foods move through the intestinal tract, the lower the incidence of disease. He noticed that communities that changed from a high-residue (high-fiber) diet to a low-residue diet also increased their intake of sugar and white-flour products. Dr. Burkitt relates the low-fiber diet and increased intake of refined carbohydrates to most of the diseases listed above as well as to the increased incidence of atherosclerosis. This information has caused the medical community to seriously reevaluate its attitude toward fiber.

As research continues, we find that fiber itself is very complex and that different types of fiber may differ in their effects on the body. Fiber consists of various materials, such as cellulose, hemicellulose, pectin, and lignins. The role that each of these plays will undoubtedly be clarified through future research, but for now it's enough to know that all types of fiber are found in a diet high in natural complex carbohydrates, such as whole grains, fruits, and vegetables. As we have seen, there are

significant benefits to be gained by increasing natural carbohydrate intake (which increases fiber intake) and reducing
refined sugars and white flours. Adding to these reasons the role
that fiber may play in the prevention of disease, this is an
obviously desirable preventive measure.

HOW FIBER HELPS US

Fiber has the capacity to hold water, which gives more substance
to the contents of the intestine. This, in turn, stimulates the walls
of the digestive tract, which aids in the elimination of waste
through the colon. Without fiber, the food in the intestines
becomes sluggish, the intestinal muscles become weak, and the
fecal matter becomes hard, slowing the time for elimination from
the body. It is speculated that this could contribute to cancer of
the colon, because of the increased amount of time that cancer-
causing agents are exposed to the colon wall. Diverticulosis
(ballooning of the colon wall), diverticulitis (infection of the
colon), hemorrhoids, and constipation are also possible results of
a low-fiber diet.

Some experts point out that these diseases may be caused by
lack of specific nutrients rather than lack of fiber. Lack of either
chromium or zinc, both essential minerals, could be the cause,
since they are also eliminated in milling. Other experts point to
the fact that high fat diets are a stronger link to cancer and heart
disease than low-fiber diets.

However, Dr. Burkitt and others who are researching fiber
make a strong point. These diseases are probably the result of a
combination of many things. If we eliminate even one of the
elements (for example, low-fiber intake), we might greatly reduce
the prevalence of disease.

A healthy diet is low in fat and high in natural carbohydrates, which means high fiber, also. It would not be wise
simply to add fiber without doing anything about reducing fat
intake. Disease, in all probability, has several causes, so it makes
sense to attack it from all angles.

Energy and Physical Performance

Ultimately, our energy is derived from the food we eat. Of the three major nutrients, carbohydrates are most important to the serious athlete. Protein, basically used for cell replacement, does not make a significant contribution to energy in metabolism. Fat is also utilized as an energy source, but it is so highly concentrated in our tissues that a well nourished body always has plenty. Carbohydrate, our most efficient energy source, can easily be depleted during strenuous exercise over a prolonged period. When carbohydrates become depleted, the body must depend on fat for its energy. Since fat is not utilized as well as carbohydrates, the performance of the athlete is reduced.

OUR LIMITING ENERGY FUEL

The intensity or speed of the activity determines which fuels—fat or carbohydrate—will dominate in supplying energy. For short, rapid events of all-out effort that last less than one or two minutes, carbohydrate is used exclusively. This is classified as *anaerobic* exercise because the energy is created without oxygen. Lifting weights or sprinting are typical examples of this high intensity activity. On the other end of the scale would be an activity such as the marathon that is less intensive but of longer duration. This is *aerobic* activity meaning that the energy occurs with oxygen. More fat will be utilized in this activity, especially as the duration increases.

As your need for oxygen increases you utilize more carbohydrate. At rest you utilize about 70% fat and only 30% carbohydrate. As you start to run you may increase your ratio to 50% carbohydrate and 50% fat.

If your intensity (speed) increases the ratio may go to 70% carbohydrate and 30% fat. Since your stores of carbohydrate are limited then you must be sure that your diet is adequate in complex carbohydrates.

Most events last only a few minutes, not long enough for an athlete to deplete the carbohydrate stores. In activities of longer duration, depletion can and often does occur. The "wall" that most marathon runners experience at about twenty miles is thought to be caused by a depletion of carbohydrates and a corresponding reliance on fat as a fuel. When a runner "hits the wall," speed and performance drop drastically.

A concern for carbohydrates is not just important in distance events. Depletion can also occur during tournament sports, where there are repeated periods of heavy exertion over a two- or three-day period.

If the "tank" isn't "full" to start with, athletes may experience the effects of carbohydrate depletion after exertion of shorter duration. This is especially common in wrestling and other sports where energy stores are depleted during weight loss and not replenished.

STORING ENERGY

Carbohydrates are stored in the body in the form of glycogen. It is estimated that a person of average size can store about 350 grams. Most glycogen is stored in the muscle tissues and liver, while some circulates in the bloodstream as glucose.

It is from the glycogen storage that energy for athletic effort is derived. As the first step in the storage process the carbohydrates are changed through digestion into glucose (blood sugar). Eventually, the glucose is stored in the muscles, where it becomes the main source of energy for exercise. It is this stored carbohydrate (glycogen) that becomes a main nutritional factor in your performance level. Storing carbohydrates takes time. It cannot be accomplished by pregame meals or by supplements taken during competition. This is why it is important for all athletes to eat a daily diet that is high in natural carbohydrates.

THE EFFECTS OF DIFFERENT DIETS
ON PERFORMANCE

Most experts in sports nutrition recommend a diet high in carbohydrates to athletes. It should be recommended to everyone! The body performs more efficiently on a high-carbohydrate diet, which increases both psychological and physiological energy. As energy expenditure goes up through extended exercises the benefits of this diet become more obvious. Let's emphasize here that we are referring only to natural carbohydrates from grains, vegetables, and fruit. The refined carbohydrates (sweets, pastries, etc.) with their high sucrose content are not recommended for serious athletes, although limited use can be tolerated.

One of the major studies demonstrating the benefits of a high-carbohydrate diet was done by the renowned physiologist Dr. Per-Olof Astrand. In this test, three diets were used. The first was a typical American diet of 50% carbohydrate, 32% fat, and 19% protein. The second was a high-fat diet of 45% fat and 54% protein. The third was a high-carbohydrate diet with 82% carbohydrate and 18% protein. Under sustained exercise conditions using a stationary bicycle, the amount of time for an athlete to reach exhaustion was measured. Those on a high-fat protein diet were able to work for a maximum of only 60 minutes! This diet, deficient in carbohydrates, is similar to the high-protein diet popular with body builders, football players, and weight lifters. Besides causing a low energy level, this diet surely increases the risk of cardiovascular disease.

Those on a normal diet fared somewhat better. Due to the added carbohydrates, they were able to maintain their training for 120 minutes. The athletes on the carbohydrate diet, however, were the ones who excelled. They tripled the performance of those on the fat-protein diet, taking 180 minutes to reach exhaustion.

The vast difference is because the athlete who eats a high-carbohydrate diet stores more carbohydrates in the muscles, so that in strenuous exercise fatigue can be delayed. Muscle biopsies have verified that there is a higher concentration of carbohydrate (glycogen) in the muscle tissue of athletes on a high-carbohydrate diet. An athlete can expect to more than double his or her storage of muscle glycogen by adhering to a high-carbohydrate diet. Those athletes who still insist on popular high-fat, high-protein diets can expect less than optimum performance, particularly in events where endurance is a factor.

TRAINING AND ITS EFFECTS
ON STORING ENERGY

Training is a major factor in top athletic performance. It is also a major factor in the ability of the body to properly convert the food eaten into energy. An athlete with a higher maximum oxygen uptake—that is, an athlete in better condition—burns fat more efficiently. If an untrained athlete attempted to hold a six-minute–mile pace with a trained athlete, he or she would quickly fall behind. The untrained athlete's higher oxygen requirement causes the body to burn carbohydrates rapidly. To this individual, the pace is more like a sprint, while to the conditioned athlete it's an easy pace to sustain.

Intensive training enhances "glycogen sparing." This is the ability of the highly trained endurance athlete to utilize more fat from the fat storage tank, thus sparing the glycogen tank and avoiding carbohydrate depletion. A well-trained athlete will have more readily available fat in the muscle tissue than an untrained athlete. Because training increases the ability of the muscles to store glycogen, a conditioned athlete can store more glycogen (energy) than an unconditioned athlete.

This phenomenon means that it is appropriate to exercise the specific muscles involved in an activity to ensure that those muscles store their maximum amount of glycogen. It is important to train at the same sport you are competing in. Runners run, wrestlers wrestle, swimmers swim, etc. Training and positive nutrition are symbiotic—one enhances the other. The right fuel enhances training, and training enhances the utilization of the fuel.

The role of fats in the diet may seem very confusing. First we say to limit fat intake. Then we say that fats are the main fuel for energy when the body is properly conditioned. This is not really a contradiction. Fat is a very important fuel to anyone, especially an athlete. However, if we ate no fat at all, our bodies would still have fat reserves, because the excess carbohydrate and protein we eat is changed to fat and stored. Through proper diet and training, the athlete stores an inexhaustible amount of fat in the muscle tissues and other parts of the body. To look at a highly trained athlete, a distance runner like Frank Shorter, for example, one would think he had no fat at all. His visible body fat (subcutaneous fat) is very low, since excess body fat would hinder his performance. He does have plenty of fat to supply his energy, however. It is simply distributed throughout his body. If this were not true, the fattest athlete would be able to run the longest!

Athletes should avoid eating fat as much as possible, since a high-fat diet has been shown to reduce endurance as well as increasing the risk of cardiovascular and degenerative diseases. Exercise alone makes a considerable contribution to the prevention of cardiovascular disease, but it is no panacea. Don't use exercise as an excuse for a high-fat diet. Your dietary fat is not significant to your energy level or your performance. Less is better.

Other factors that have a negative effect on performance as a result of a high-fat diet are:

1. *A high fat diet that is very low in carbohydrates can cause ketosis.* With fat as the main fuel to supply energy, the body does not function too well. When the body's premium fuel, carbo-hydrate, is eliminated, fat is burned. However, fat does not burn as efficiently as carbohydrate, and a residue, ketones (a product of fat metabolism), builds up in the bloodstream. Ketosis reduces the endurance level, reduces mental awareness, and reduces overall performance level. People on high-fat diets often complain of weakness, dizziness, and a lack of energy, signs of ketosis. Heavy exercise intensifies these effects.

2. *Fat can reduce the oxygen supply to the cells.* Dr. Meyer Friedman, director of the National Heart, Lung, and Blood Institute, found that a meal high in fat reduces cellular oxygen. During digestion excess fat passes into the lymphatic system. Within several hours, the fat enters the bloodstream, where it coats the red blood cells. This causes the red blood cells (which carry oxygen) to "clump" or stick together. "Clumping" reduces the flow of these oxygen-carrying red cells through the small capillaries. The end result is a reduced oxygen supply to the cells. This reduced oxygen supply to the heart muscle could cause angina (chest pain) in heart patients. Whether it actually reduces the oxygen supply to the active muscles of athletes is speculative, but it may be another supportive consideration for a low-fat diet.

When nutritionists or doctors say not to worry about getting enough fat in the diet, they are giving you sound advice. They know that no matter how hard we try to avoid fat, we will still get at least 10% of the calories in our diet in the form of fat. That amount is more than sufficient to meet anyone's needs, especially an athlete's. Dr. Joan Ullyot, a long-distance runner, concisely states the best position on fats when she says, "The distinction between active, 'trained-on' fat and passive, 'eaten-on' fat is very important." Only the former is useful. Otherwise, the best eater would be the best runner.

CARBOHYDRATE LOADING

At this point we are well aware that an adequate supply of carbohydrate is essential for maximum performance and that carbohydrate is stored in the muscles and liver as glycogen, then supplied to the working muscle. If we can increase the amount of stored glycogen, then we can reduce the onset of fatigue and loss of energy during prolonged endurance events. Research has shown that through diet manipulation, we can almost triple the amount of glycogen stored in the exercised muscle.

This is accomplished with a diet and workout adjustment referred to as "carbohydrate loading" during the week prior to competition. The first three days of this program involve a very high fat-high protein diet accompanied by exhaustive workouts. This tends to deplete the muscular stores of glycogen, causing fatigue and reduced performance during training. For the next three days the athlete eats a very high carbohydrate diet and rests. This ensures a super-saturation of muscle glycogen. This technique is similar to squeezing as much water as possible out of a sponge (depletion phase), then placing the sponge in water and soaking up the maximum possible amount of water (loading phase).

SHOULD YOU CARBOHYDRATE LOAD?

In endurance events lasting more than 1½ hours, it has been shown that runners who "load" are able to delay the onset of fatigue and hold their pace toward the end of the race much better than the "nonloaders." It is important to point out that for sports which require 1½ hours of sustained exercise or less, carbohydrate loading probably serves no purpose, as long as normal glycogen stores are adequate.

The practice of carbohydrate loading for super-saturation of glycogen is basically unsound. The first phase, which includes a high-fat, high-protein diet, is not nutritionally desirable. This is the very diet cardiologists and nutritionists recommend that we avoid, because of its relationship to heart and vascular disease. There is some question whether this phase is really important. Some research suggests that the high-fat, high-protein phase can be omitted altogether with little change in performance.

The other phase of the diet is the loading of carbohydrates. Many athletes incorrectly select sweets and other junk foods (cake, pie, sodas, ice cream, pastry, etc.) as an enjoyable way to "load up." They think "load" means to eat all they can. Some trainers and coaches even recommend this practice. But an athlete stuffed with too much food, especially junk food, is not going to perform well.

Under super-loading practices, the depletion phase usually lasts two to three days, with a daily carbohydrate intake of only 60 grams. At this low level, the athlete is taking in only about 10% carbohydrate. The procedure requires an exhaustive workout prior to depletion and again prior to the loading phase. During this period the athlete will become very fatigued, irritable, and quite possibly nauseous, as a result of the low carbohydrate intake. His or her times will be considerably reduced during this period and, coupled with the negative physiological responses, the athlete's psychological attitude may be negatively affected as competition approaches.

As practiced, this diet actually becomes the very one that health and nutrition experts recommend we avoid. Besides the cardiovascular risk there is some indication that this diet may be deficient in vitamins and minerals. It is also important to consider the effects on athletes predisposed to diabetes before instituting this diet in a training program.

A HEALTHIER WAY
TO CARBOHYDRATE LOAD

Recent studies have raised questions about the effectiveness of super-saturation of carbohydrates for endurance events. The more widely accepted method is simply an increase in carbohydrates and the elimination of the depletion phase with its associated high-fat diet. This would involve a depletion workout approximately three days prior to competition, followed by a high-carbohydrate diet (80% of total calories) during the following three days.

Since athletes should be on a high-carbohydrate diet all the time, this slight increase should not require a major change in eating habits. During those last three days you should reduce your training load to a minimum level and rest the body to ensure a higher glycogen store in the muscles.

Remember that carbohydrate "load" doesn't mean to eat more food and stuff yourself. It simply means to change the proportions of carbohydrates, fat, and protein. Don't make the mistake many athletes do and use it as an excuse to stuff yourself with cake, pie, soda, beer, and other refined products.

CARBOHYDRATES FOR EVENTS
LASTING LESS THAN
ONE AND ONE-HALF HOURS

Carbohydrate loading is not necessary for athletes involved in activities that last less than 1½ hours. Training itself will increase the muscle glycogen stores if the basic diet is high in carbohydrates. A basic diet of 60 to 70% carbohydrates will ensure that adequate carbohydrates are available during competition. The "average" person is capable of storing about 350 grams of carbohydrate, which is 1,400 calories of stored energy. Even in exhaustive sustained exercise, it would take over one hour to deplete these stores. Running continuously for 60 minutes at a five-minute-per-mile pace would burn 1,200 calories. A wrestler working continuously for 60 minutes would burn about 900 calories. Most events are intermittent and require considerably fewer calories. Remember, too, that at lower activity levels fat is being burned for some of the energy requirements.

The main point to remember with regard to loading is that a well-trained athlete will store more glycogen. If you maintain a high-carbohydrate diet during training you will be able to tolerate higher levels of training, which in turn enables you to store more glycogen. Being more oxygen efficient, you will also burn more fat, thus "sparing" your limited muscle glycogen.

The new interest in biathlons and triathlons will present new dietary challenges to sports medicine. Their longer time-frame, which can be in excess of nine hours, makes proper diet even more meaningful. Since a triathlon involves different activities (running—swimming—biking), I would be sure to do a depletion workout in each activity to deplete the glycogen stores in the specific muscles used in each event. I'm sure we will see more research in this area in the future.

Questions and Answers

Q: *Is too much sugar related to hyeractivity in children?*
A: That's really never been proven. However, there is some indication that low blood sugar may trigger hyperactivity in susceptible children. Most of us are not aware of the huge quantity of sugar children consume. Many youngsters down over 1,000 soft drinks a year.

Q: *Why do manufactures take the germ and bran out of bread during milling?*
A: The bran and the germ clog up the steel rollers that mill flour, and the flour goes rancid faster with the germ in. By getting rid of both, manufacturers can make a product that is easier to market

and has long shelf life. It's great for the bread manufacturer, but not for our health. The bran and the germ are sold to livestock feeders as animal feed. The animals stay very healthy on all the vitamins, minerals, and fiber found in the germ and bran, but we would be better off if they were included in our diet.

Q: *When I have a candy bar or soft drink I get a surge of "energy." What's wrong with that?*
A: The energy is temporary and is usually followed by a drop in energy due to low blood sugar. This makes you crave something sweet and the cycle starts all over. You overwork your pancreas, take in excess sugar, get excess calories, which can lead to obesity, and get no nutrients. You are flooding your engine with sugar.

Q: *What's a better choice?*
A: Anything without refined sugar! If you're active, whole fruit—such as banana or orange—is fine.

Q: *I thought diabetics were supposed to eat a lot of high-protein foods like meat, cheese, and eggs.*
A: That has changed. The new recommendation for diabetics is similar to the natural carbohydrate diet we all should eat. Some modification is needed for the diabetic, but the high-fat and high-protein diet is no longer ideal. Refined sugar products should be greatly reduced.

Q: *Is honey better to use than sugar as a sweetener?*
A: Yes and no. Honey does have some vitamins and minerals, but not enough to make much difference. It's a good substitute for refined sugar, but keep it down. You can live just fine without any sugar in your diet.

Q: *But I thought you had to have some sugar in your diet.*
A: No. Not refined sugar. The only sugar you need is glucose, which is derived from complex carbohydrates.

Q: *Then it's bad to eat any sugar?*
A: No. A small amount will do no harm. A treat now and then is okay. It's what you eat regularly that is important, not what you have once in a while.

Q: *I've heard that nuts and seeds are a good energy snack.*
A: No. That idea came about because nuts and seeds are part of the plant kingdom and are thought of as carbohydrates. Most nuts and seeds are 70% fat. Since they have vitamins, minerals, and protein they contribute to your nutrition, but consider them as part of your total fat intake and don't overdo a good thing.

Q: *Our health-food store carries several types of raw sugar. Which is best?*
A: There is no raw sugar sold in the United States! What you refer to as raw is actually sucrose, just like white sugar. It probably has a little molasses in it, but that adds an insignificant amount of vitamins and minerals, only changing the color to brown. All of these sugars are 87% to 97% refined white sugar. They cost more without accomplishing more.

Q: *What should I use as a sweetener?*
A: Nothing. Rather than look for all the ways to substitute for sugar, such as using honey, molasses, or date sugar, just avoid sugars as much as possible. You might try fresh fruit (like bananas and strawberries) with your cereal rather than sugar. Addiction is hard to break.

Q: *But health-food stores sell all kinds of products that substitute honey for sugar. Aren't these better?*
A: Yes, if you don't use them very much. If you substitute equal amounts of honey for refined sugar, you haven't made much of a change for the better. Health-food stores are run by *people*, just like markets. They mean well but get caught up in the greed for profit. I've found many health-food products loaded with sugar, fats, and additives. Read labels and ask questions!

Q: *Can you become addicted to sugar?*
A: Yes. The immediate effect of sugar is an energy surge, which gradually gives way to fatigue. Like drugs, this encourages consumption of more sugar for that temporary high.

Q: *How can I tell if I'm diabetic or hypoglycemic?*
A: You can't! But a medical doctor with experience in diabetes can. One test you would be given would be a 6-hour glucose tolerance test. If you experience any adverse symptoms, you would do well to contact your doctor for tests and evaluation.

Q: *How about saccharin as a sugar substitute?*
A: Saccharin is not a food. Not much is known about its effect on the body, but research indicates it may be carcinogenic. It may well be banned by the time you read this! I'd stay away from it. Small amounts of sugar or honey in your coffee aren't going to make you fat.

Q: *What do you suggest I do with all the candy my kids collect on Hallowe'en?*
A: Educate them. Tell them it's bad for them and why. Take a few apples and oranges out of the bag and dump the "junk" on the floor. Tell them they can eat all they want, but what is left gets thrown out in the morning. They will love the idea at first, but in the morning they will definitely be associating sickness with junk food! Remember, you're trying to fight the multi-billion-dollar sugar industry.

Q: *Did you say there is sugar in hot dogs?*
A: Yes. Most processed meats have added sugar. Read the labels.

Q: *I've been told that the sugar from fruit is no different than table sugar because they both contain the same sugars, glucose and fructose. Is that true?*
A: They do contain the same sugars, but they are not interchangeable. Fruit differs from table sugar in several ways. The sugar in fruit is associated with fiber, is diluted in a large volume of water, and is mixed with many vitamins and minerals essential to health. Sugar from fruit will be much better tolerated by the body as an energy source. Table sugar supplies only energy without the positive characteristics of fruit.

Q: *I like the idea of increasing my fiber, but I'm worried I won't get the correct amount or type. What do your suggest?*
A: Make some commonsense changes. Add a little bran to cereals, muffins, and bread. Also, eat more whole grains, whole fruits, raw vegetables, and legumes. Concentrate on eliminating refined sugar and white-flour products as well.

Q: *Does a high-fiber diet have a positive effect on diabetes?*
A: Dr. Margaret J. Albrink of West Virginia University showed that a high-fiber diet provoked an insulin response less than one-half that provoked by a formula diet. (What that means is

that the blood sugar level did not go up rapidly on the high-fiber diet.) Both diets had equal amounts of fat, protein, and carbohydrate.

Q: *How do I know I'm getting enough fiber?*
A: If you're eating a diet similar to the one we recommend—high in natural carbohydrates—your intake is probably adequate. On the other hand, if your diet is still high in animal products, processed foods, sugar, and white flour, it's probably too low in fiber. A nutritionist once said, "Frequency and flotation are a good indicator." That means that how often you have a bowel movement and how high it floats indicate whether your diet is sufficient in fiber—the more often and higher, the better!

Q: *Is increasing fiber a better way to lower the cholesterol level than by reducing fats in the diet?*
A: A high-fiber diet certainly helps, but it's probably only one factor in controlling the cholesterol level. For example, if you had a high cholesterol level of 300 milligrams and reduced it 10%, by increasing the fiber content of the diet, you would lower it only to 270 milligrams. That still leaves you in a high-risk area for heart disease. The optimum diet would lower both fat and cholesterol intake, while increasing fiber.

Q: *You mentioned that a high-fiber diet might reduce cancer of the colon. Could you explain that?*
A: It is speculated that refined sugar and flour in *low-residue* diets promote a type of colon bacteria that can change bile salts into carcinogenic substances. The low-residue diet moves slowly through the colon, where the tissue of the colon is exposed to the carcinogens for a longer time. High-fiber diets promote the growth of different bacteria that don't form carcinogens.

Q: *How can more fiber have an effect on obesity and weight loss?*
A: Fiber fills you up faster without high calorie intake. Let's take two examples: An apple has about 70 calories, and it is a high-fiber food, as well as being an excellent carbohydrate. In contrast, a Milky Way candy bar may also fill you up, but it has 240 calories. How fast and how many of each can you eat? Most of us could eat two candy bars in a short time. That's almost 500

calories, which is easily one-fourth of most people's daily calorie need. It would take *eight apples* to provide 500 calories.

Think you're full? Try this. Eat five pieces of white bread and note how full you feel. Later, eat five pieces of stoneground whole-grain bread. You will find it difficult to finish the whole-grain bread. If you get full on fewer calories, but actually eat more food, it is better for you!

Q: *How much fiber do we need?*
A: We don't know exactly how much we need. In the studies done by Dr. Dennis Burkitt, mentioned earlier, the dietary fiber intake was between 25 and 35 grams a day. Approaching this amount may be a reasonable goal. Don't be overly concerned with numbers, though. Including high-fiber foods and reducing your intake of fats and refined sugars will do the job.

Q: *What foods should I eat to increase my dietary fiber?*
A: No particular food is best, because each acts differently. Bran, the fiber of wheat, has been highly touted by popular diet books. Bran can hold five times its weight in water; but that doesn't make it the only fiber that's important. *All* natural carbohydrates contain some fiber. Whole-grain breads and cereals, bran cereals, wheat germ, dried peas and beans, fresh fruit with skins, and raw vegetables are all high in fiber and are all good foods to include in your diet.

Q: *Can you get too much fiber?*
A: Yes. Some popular nutrition books suggest taking 10 tablespoons of bran a day, while maintaining your typical American diet! This would undoubtedly cause diarrhea, which will interfere with your absorption of vitamins and minerals. People love the idea that they can eat a junky, refined, high-fat diet and just add 10 tablespoons of bran to be healthy. Don't believe it!

Q: *How does fiber affect heart disease?*
A: Fiber may lower serum cholesterol. Studies done by Dr. Kritchevsky and J.A. Story, which appeared in the *Journal of Nutrition* in 1974, have shown that increasing fiber in the diet can cause a decrease in serum cholesterol levels of about 10%.

Cholesterol is excreted from the body by way of bile salts. The liver turns cholesterol into bile salts and secretes it into the intestine, where much of it binds with certain fibers found in the residue and is carried out of the body. Interestingly, the fibers of legumes and apples seem to be very effective, while bran, the most popularly used fiber, *has no effect in lowering the cholesterol level.*

Q: *If athletes in short, fast events used 100% carbohydrate, wouldn't they need more carbohydrate in their diet?*
A: No. Even though the athlete is using 100% carbohydrate the duration (time) of the activity is too short to deplete his stores of carbohydrate.

Q: *What if you did successive short workouts over a prolonged time?*
A: Then total carbohydrate stores become more important. The safest measure is for all athletes to eat a higher-than-average carbohydrate diet.

Q: *What if you run out of carbohydrate?*
A: You will burn fat. This means you must slow your intensity since fat burns slowly. Protein and glycerol will be converted to glucose to maintain the nervous system, but little will be available for muscle energy requirements.

Q: *Can I store excessive amounts of carbohydrate, possibly enough to compete at a very high level for a long time?*
A: Although an individual can triple storage of carbohydrates through proper diet and training, there is still a point of diminishing returns. Through training the body can learn to utilize fats more efficiently, thus sparing carbohydrate stores. Until research can come up with other ways of increasing our utilization of fat, the 80%-carbohydrate diet is your best bet.

Q: *Does it help to switch to a high-carbohydrate diet the night before competition?*
A: Yes. But not much. Any diet adjustment that increases the complex carbohydrate intake is worthwhile. For the best results start at least 48 hours prior to competition.

Q: *Am I correct in assuming that as I increase my speed (intensity), I burn more cabohydrate?*
A: Yes. And if you reduce your speed and increase duration you burn more fat, thus "sparing" your limited carbohydrate stores.

Q: *How can I go faster and still avoid running out of carbohydrate fuel?*
A: Through training. Eating a high-carbohydrate diet is the first step in storing more energy. Through training your oxygen utilization increases, which means your body burns less carbohydrate and more fat without a reduction in performance. Highly conditioned athletes don't burn off their carbohydrate stores, and it seems that they burn fat more efficiently.

Q: *Why is it important to exercise the specific muscles for carbohydrate storage?*
A: Because the muscles used store the most carbohydrate. A swimmer would store more glycogen (stored carbohydrate) in his arms, and a runner would store more in his legs. Be sure to spend a good amount of your conditioning time doing the specific activity you will perform.

Q: *One of our football players is on a high-protein–high-fat diet. Could this be the cause of his obvious fatigue?*
A: Yes. He doesn't have enough carbohydrate to function at a high level. His fatigue is the result of trying to train and compete on a low-energy fuel. He'll do great if he just sits on the bench, but don't expect any spurts of energy on the field.

Q: *Can I run out of fat as an energy source?*
A: For all practical purposes—no. Fat is so highly concentrated that even the skinniest athlete has more than enough. Remember, too, that every excess calorie of protein and carbohydrate is converted to fat!

5
VITAMINS
AND MINERALS

The Function
of Vitamins and Minerals

Vitamins and minerals can be viewed as nutrients, required in very small amounts, that enhance our health. They can't supply energy to the body as carbohydrates do, nor build and replace tissue as protein does, but they are still very important. Specifically, vitamins act as a catalyst on the food we eat in much the same manner that a spark can ignite a fire in the presence of oxygen and fuel. They are important regulators of literally thousands of chemical reactions that affect our growth, function, and metabolism.

Contrary to popular belief, no one vitamin or mineral is really much more important than another. For example, almost everyone knows that vitamins A and D are important vitamins, but lesser-known nutrients like folic acid, selenium, or zinc are equally important to optimum health.

Minerals are inorganic substances involved with many vital functions of the body. They give structure to bones and teeth, maintain a neutral acid base of blood tissue, control heart and muscle contraction, control normal nerve responses, and perform an array of other equally important tasks.

Vitamins and minerals are referred to as "micro" nutrients because we require such small amounts of them compared to the "macro" nutrients—carbohydrates, protein, and fat. We can easily consume 100 grams of carbohydrate in a normal diet, while that same diet may yield only a few milligrams of a specific vitamin or mineral. This balance seems to be consistent with nature's balance.

Food: Our Source of Nutrients

Wholesome, natural food is the best source of vitamins and minerals. "Wholesome" and "natural" are the key words! Ideally, we should select foods that are as close to their natural state as possible. Unfortunately, most of the food readily available to us is highly processed and lacks the balance of vitamins and minerals characteristic of natural foods.

Poor selection of nutritious food is probably the paramount reason that most government studies show widespread vitamin and mineral deficiencies in the United States. The fast-paced American life-style lends itself to convenience foods, which are highly processed and are usually very poorly balanced in nutrients. The common example of "milled grains," which we discussed earlier, is only one of many examples. The enrichment or fortification of processed food does help; but since it does not replace the total nutrients that are removed in the milling, the food loses its balance of nutrients that are essential to optimum health. With the general public subject to a barrage of advertising and promotion for fast food, instant food, convenience food, and, now, "fun food," it's not surprising that many people find it difficult to eat nutritiously. The first step in increasing your vitamin and mineral intake is to select as many wholesome, natural products as you can; but even then you will find there are no guarantees.

Food will always be our main source of vitamins and minerals. Nature can supply all the nutrients in a balanced level in a mixed diet composed of wholesome foods.

In recent years, the quality of our food supply has been questioned by research scientists. Our increased use of convenience food in the form of canned and packaged food has increased our potential for vitamin and mineral deficiencies. Even fresh vegetables and fruits may not contain the amount of nutrients we assume they do. There are many factors that affect the nutrient content of fresh food. Growing conditions, storage, shipping, and transportation time can significantly affect the vitamin and mineral content of fruits and vegetables. If we look at the *Nutrient Value of American Foods,* Agriculture Handbook No. 456, we see that a common orange contains about 85 milligrams of vitamin C. Even though that amount may be typical it does not necessarily mean that *all* oranges contain 85 milligrams. In his book, *Your Personal Vitamin Profile* (New York: William Morrow Co., 1982), Dr. Michael Colgan tested various oranges from local markets. Not too surprisingly, he found that the vitamin C content varied from a high of 180 milligrams to a low of zero. Obviously, if the orange you happen to eat contains no vitamin C, you will need to get it from some other food. Canned and frozen foods can vary greatly in nutrient content, also. In processing, vegetables are scalded to destroy the enzymes that would cause decomposition. Remaining enzymes are deactivated by freezing and sterilization, which can reduce the vitamin and mineral content.

Dr. Henry A. Schroeder, of Dartmouth Medical School, has done some of the most significant research on the vitamin and mineral content of food. He has found a wide degree of nutrient loss in both canned and frozen foods. Here are just a few examples: frozen vegetables lost 36% to 44% of vitamin B_6; canned vegetables, 57% to 77% of vitamin B_6; and canned tomatoes, 80% of the zinc. Freezing can destroy half the B vitamins. Even without the problems associated with production of food, the consumer does a considerable amount of damage. Cooking and food preparation in the home can destroy 54% of the nutrient value of food, and probably the same can be said for much of the food we eat in restaurants. Boiling is the least desirable way to cook. Large amounts of water and exposure to heat and oxygen contribute to nutrient depletion. A vegetable steamer might be a good investment to help reduce the vitamin and mineral loss in cooked vegetables.

A word about "organic produce" would probably be worthwhile here. If you're planning to switch to organic produce to get more vitamins and minerals, free of pollutants, you may be wasting your time and money. There are no reliable studies to support the theory that organic foods are higher in vitamin and mineral content. It is true that soil depletion can reduce the mineral (not vitamin) content of produce, but the use of "organic" fertilizers is no guarantee of a higher mineral content. Chemical fertilizers may be an even better way to replace any mineral depletion that may occur in plant foods. As far as pesticides are concerned, actual tests do not show a difference between the pesticide content of organic produce and the supermarket variety. Just to prove the point, ask the manager of a local health-food store to guarantee in writing that the produce is higher in vitamins and minerals and less contaminated with pesticides than the same produce sold in the supermarket. Don't hold your breath!

Our discussion so far has shown that just eating food isn't a gurarantee of good nutrition. Quite simply, we have changed the food we eat. In an effort to feed an expanding population, to make eating a convenience, and to keep the cost down we have changed the structure of our diets. It's just too easy (or too convenient) to select the wrong foods in a society that lives on predominantly processed food. Keeping your diet simple, selecting a variety of fresh wholesome products, and proper preparation will help to maintain the vitamin and mineral content of your diet at a higher level.

Should You Take Supplements?

If you think politics is controversial, then you haven't seen anything yet! Nutritionists will agree on almost any areas of nutrition and health except the debate over whether one should take vitamin and mineral supplements. Supplementing the diet with nutrients is the most controversial area of nutrition. Unfortunately, you, the consumer, are caught in the middle, because some very eminent and respected scientific authorities line up on each side of the controversy. The main thrust of the controversy goes like this: Those opposed to supplements feel that a balanced diet, correctly selected, will supply all the vitamins and minerals you require. They also, quite accurately, point out that you can get too much of a good thing in a supplement (too much of a vitamin or mineral). On the other side are those experts who believe that the mixed diet selected by most people will not supply the correct balance of nutrients for optimum health. If you're waiting for me to take your hand and guide you into the light of knowledge, you'll have a long wait! Like many health professionals, I'm not really sure who is right. (I'll admit it, most won't.)

Frankly, I think the controversy is too extreme. In support of the knowledgeable scientists who are against supplements, I think eating a balanced diet *is* the best way to get your nutrients. But in actual practice few people eat the mythical "balanced diet." These scientists also assume that all the food selections you make will contain adequate amounts of all the nutrients required for good health. As we have seen, such is not always the case. More importantly, I'm not sure a lot of people will eat a good diet even if they know what one is.

We actually supplement our diet all the time. Many processed foods are "enriched" or "fortified" with vitamins and minerals. Yet no one attacks the food processors for pushing products such as enriched cereals, pastries, imitation fruit drinks, desserts, and breads as good sources of vitamins and minerals. The makers of some products even advertise that you can get 100% of your R.D.A. in one serving! That's a poor trade-off for the sugar, fat, and salt that many of these products contain.

As with most things in life, you will have to make your decision alone. To help (or confuse) you, you may want to read two books with opposing views. In support of nutritional supplementation Dr. Colgan's book, *Your Personal Vitamin Profile,* is excellent. A good book against supplementation is *Vitamins and Health Foods: The Great American Hustle,* by Victor D. Herbert and Stephen Barrett (Philadelphia, PA: G. F. Stickley, 1981). Dr. Victor Herbert is a highly respected nutritional researcher from the State University of New York.

The best I can do here is to give you some guidelines. Let's look at some of the factors that may affect your need for vitamins and minerals.

We are not all the same. The Food and Nutrition board of the National Academy of Science establishes the recommended daily allowance (R.D.A.) for each nutrient. The R.D.A. is an estimate (based on research) of the amount of each vitamin and mineral we should get in our daily diet. These are not meant to be requirements. The individual requirements for vitamins and minerals can vary greatly from individual to individual. Dr. Roger J. Williams emphasized this important point in his classic 1963 book *Bio-Chemical Individuality.* Dr. Williams found that some people may require as much as ten times the amount of a single vitamin than the amount assumed. Of course, determining who needs more or less of specific nutrients is going to be a challenge to nutritional scientists in the future. By individual evaluation we may one day be able to determine the nutrient requirement based on bio-chemical individuality.

Environmental Antagonists That Create Deficiencies

Besides our genetic differences, which cause variations in our vitamin and mineral requirements, we have other factors that affect our ability to absorb and utilize nutrients as well as increase our need for specific nutrients. These are the environmental antagonists. Some are under our control and some are not. Alcohol consumption, smoking, dieting, stress, pollution, medication, surgery, age, exercise, and a host of other factors affect our nutritional needs. Let's look at a few:

Alcohol consumption: A high level of alcohol use (about three or more drinks daily) increases our chances of vitamin and mineral deficiencies. Among heavy drinkers the need for many of the B vitamins, folacin, zinc, magnesium, and vitamin A is increased. Damage to the liver resulting from excessive alcohol use interferes with the absorption and storage of vitamins and increases our need for vitamins to metabolize the alcohol itself.

Smoking: There is no safe level of smoking. I think all health professionals would label smoking the single worst contaminant put into our bodies. Besides its well-known contribution to lung cancer and heart disease, smoking is linked to many other diseases, such as ulcers, bronchitis, and emphysema, and is associated with other cancers besides lung cancer. It suppresses the immune system, which is one of the body's main defenders against disease. Smoking also increases the need for vitamins. The vitamin C content of the blood is lower in smokers than in nonsmokers.

Dieting: Who hasn't gone on a diet? The simple act of reducing calories proportionately reduces your intake of vitamins and minerals. Anyone who stays on a restricted diet for too long will require additional supplements.

Surgery: Surgery, as well as other illnesses, increases our need for nutrients. This is a very neglected area of hospital food services.

Age: As we get older our ability to absorb nutrients from the digestive tract decreases. This is especially true of the water soluble vitamins B and C. Older people also tend to limit the variety and quantity of foods they eat and thus ingest fewer nutrients.

Drugs: The use of oral contraceptives, prescription drugs, and illegal drugs can all increase the need for vitamins and minerals. Mainly, they interfere with absorption. Antibiotics destroy the intestinal bacteria that synthesize many of our B vitamins.

Refined sugars: Refined sugar itself does not contain the nutrients required for its own metabolism. If your diet is high in refined-sugar products you may have an increased need for the B vitamins because the excessive sugar may rob the B vitamins from other foods in the diet.

Pollution: The environmental awareness of the sixties made us all a little bit more enlightened about the effect of pollutants on our health. We are exposed to a number of pollutants from the air we breathe, our food, and a multitude of industrial toxic wastes that find their way into our bodies. They come in all forms: cosmetics, cigarette smoke, petroleum products, insecticides, etc. Many of these pollutants can destroy nutrients and cause certain illnesses and disease. Several vitamins and minerals, especially vitamins C and E, and the minerals selenium, zinc, and iron, have been shown to reduce the toxic effect of many pollutants.

Many of these conditions are avoidable. Many are not. Reducing alcohol consumption, avoiding smoking, and increasing your amount of exercise instead of drastically limiting your calorie intake for weight control are better choices than just loading up on vitamin supplements. The important thing to remember is that you must evaluate your personal environment to determine how adequate your diet is in maintaining your nutrient requirements.

The Importance of Balancing Nutrients

If you think you can just load up on specific vitamins and minerals to protect you, then you are sadly mistaken. Nutrients act in combination with other nutrients. There are literally thousands of interactions. Just taking vitamin C because you smoke may do nothing for you if you're not getting a balance of all the nutrients that work with vitamin C. If you were to take calcium, for example, because you're worried about getting osteoporosis, the calcium would be useless if your body did not also contain an adequate amount of vitamin D. The use of single-nutrient supplementation is one of the most abused areas of nutrition. Vitamin hucksters are constantly telling us how this or that nutrient can prevent this or that condition. Athletes will take many times more vitamin E than is reasonable because someone told them it increases endurance. Even if it does affect endurance (which is doubtful), it doesn't do it alone!

An Attitude Toward Supplements

If you do take supplements, take them for the right reasons. Too many people take supplements instead of improving their eating habits and assume that supplements will compensate for a poor diet. They may help, but they surely will not lead to optimum health. Another common practice is to play doctor and start taking single nutrients to prevent or cure diseases or ailments.

Your first and most important objective is to improve your diet and adjust your living pattern in such a manner that you avoid the environmental antagonists we mentioned previously. Your use of supplements should support your positive nutritional changes by lending some insurance to your diet. In this regard you should look for a supplement that is balanced in all the vitamins and minerals. Leave the use of megavitamin therapy and disease control to medical doctors competent and knowledgeable in nutritional therapy. This will not only save you money but it will reduce the risk of getting too much of one nutrient, which could possibly cause a deficiency in other nutrients and inadvertently lead to poor health.

Megavitamin and Megamineral Supplementation

The indiscriminate use of megavitamin and megamineral supplementation is of great concern to doctors and researchers. A small group of scientists is studying the possible benefits of using very large doses of supplements to correct some medical problems. They have experienced some success in the areas of mental illness and gross dietary deficiencies.

Most experts look at very large doses (doses extremely above the normal intake) of vitamins and minerals as drug therapy. Under the supervision of nutritionally qualified doctors, this may have considerable merit both in the correction and in the prevention of disease.

However, promoters have now gotten into the picture and have started suggesting that megatherapy is good for everyone! That could very well turn out to be a dangerous practice, since no one in nutritional research can guarantee the safety of such a practice when it is not medically supervised. It's quite possible we can get too much of a good thing!

A case in point, which has received considerable attention, is the use of vitamin C. Linus Pauling, the Nobel Prize winner, suggested several years ago that the average intake of vitamin C should be about 10 grams a day. When you consider that the R.D.A. is only 60 milligrams, you can appreciate the furor that developed in the scientific community. He is suggesting we take 166 times the R.D.A. Had Pauling not been such a distinguished scientist, he would definitely have been labeled a quack! Dr. Pauling does present some convincing evidence for his theory (*Vitamin C and the Common Cold* by Linus Pauling), and in time he could be proven correct. He has demonstrated that megadoses of vitamin C boost the effectiveness of the immune system. However, this is still theory, not proven fact. On the other side of the coin, Dr. Gerhard N. Schrauzer of the University of California, San Diego, found that excessive intake of vitamin C (over 3,000 milligrams a day) over a prolonged time alters the regulating system which speeds the breakdown and excretion of vitamin C.

It is well documented that excessive intake of the fat-soluble vitamins, especially A and D, may be toxic. Unlike the water-soluble vitamins, the B complex (all the B vitamins) and vitamin C, the fat-soluble vitamins are stored in the body. The potential for toxicity is then much greater.

What is best for the average person? To take a supplement above the R.D.A., especially vitamins B and C is probably safe. But to take very large doses may in time prove dangerous. The supposed need for most of the B vitamins is only a few milligrams. To take ten and twenty times that amount may be safe. To take 200 times that amount is unwarranted in light of present research and because of possible dangerous effects not yet recognized.

GUIDELINES FOR USING SUPPLEMENTS

1. Avoid large doses, especially of the fat-soluble vitamins A, D, E, and K.
2. Don't take separate supplements of the B vitamins. They function best in their complex (all together). Separate doses should be therapeutically supervised by a doctor.
3. Larger doses of vitamins B and C are relatively safe, but don't overdo it.
4. Toxic level: pay close attention to the toxicity levels of the vitamins and minerals listed at the end of the chapter. *Do not take these megadose levels unless you're under a doctor's care for specific treatment.*

The Role of Supplements in the Athlete's Diet

Since sports began, athletes have been looking for a magic pill that will increase endurance and stamina and make them win. It is not uncommon to see athletes fall prey to wishful thinking and stuff themselves with B_{15}, bee pollen, or any number of other nutrients in the hope that they will become instant champions. The fact that no supportive research defends this practice does not seem to slow the trend. Promoters know all too well how to play on the psyche of the serious athlete. If they can put some doubt in the mind of the athlete about his or her ability to win without this or that supplement, sales will go up.

The major problem among athletes is that they look at supplements as an aid—that is, as a substance that will increase their energy or performance. As delightful as that idea may sound, it just isn't sound. The idea is, of course, typical of our society. Everyone has been brought up with the concept that instant energy or instant happiness is only a pill away. We are conditioned that way, which is unfortunate.

There was a time (perhaps this is still true) when musicians felt that drugs gave them the inspiration to be creative. Sidney Cohen, a drug researcher, commented "Creativity is 90% perspiration and only 10% inspiration." Sports are very similar. Perspiration from hard training is the major component of success. Good nutrition, with or without all of the supplements available, cannot produce champions if athletes don't train hard!

Do Vitamins and Minerals
Improve Performance?

I have stated before that nutrients work best synergistically; that is, they work best together. Most of the studies done with vitamins have dealt only with the effect of a single nutrient on performance. Dr. Michal Colgan, of the Colgan Institute of Nutritional Science in Carlsbad, California, says that single-nutrient studies on performance cannot always show a positive result because there is no assurance that the rest of the nutrient complex is available. Secondly, it takes time, at least six months, before the physiological effect of a supplement might appear. Short-term studies are worthless. In spite of this flaw in the research, there is some support for the increased need for the vitamin B complex and vitamin C in endurance training. The additional calories that endurance atheltes consume will probably supply this additional requirement of vitamin B complex and vitamin C *if* those calories are made up of food high in these nutrients. If the additional calories are refined sugars, then it is more probable that a deficiency can occur. Dr. Colgan has tested both runners and weight lifters using a complete vitamin and mineral supplement designed for the individual. He presents convincing evidence based on double-blind* studies that the

---

Double Blind Study: A study in which there is a control group and an experimental group. Neither the scientist or those being tested know which group is receiving the supplement or the placebo.

athletes in his study improved their overall performance with the aid of a balanced supplement. Unlike the short-term studies, Dr. Colgan's experiment ran six months. I'm sure sports medicine will hear more from Dr. Colgan in the future. If we are able to improve performance with vitamins and minerals, it will no doubt be with a balanced supplement combined with a nutritious diet. Only then will the total human machine improve physiologically to achieve an optimum state of health.

Suggested Maintenance Level for a Vitamin and Mineral Supplement

The following suggested supplement is intended as a guide to help you select adequate amounts of each nutrient, amounts above the R.D.A. but well below the megadose levels. The term "maintenance range" does not imply that the higher level is better. Rather, it is intended as a limit. For most people staying at the lower end of the scale will be more than adequate for maintenance purposes.

Following the suggested supplement is a list of the vitamins and minerals with a brief statement of their functions in the body and some good food sources. Pay special attention to the "toxic level" of each nutrient, and stay well below that amount.

NUTRIENT	MAINTENANCE RANGE
Vitamin A	1,000–3,000 mcg.* RE**
Vitamin B₁ (Thiamine)	2–25 mg.
Vitamin B₂ (Riboflavin)	2–25 mg.
Vitamin B₃ (Niacin)	20–100 mg.
Vitamin B₅ (Pantothenic Acid)	5–25 mg.
Vitamin B₆ (Pyridoxine)	5–25 mg.
Vitamin B₁₂ (Cyanocobalamin)	5–25 mcg.
Folic Acid	400 mcg.
Biotin	2–5 mg.
Inositol	100–200 mg.
Para-Amino-Benzoic Acid (PABA)	25–50 mg.

NUTRIENT (continued)	MAINTENANCE RANGE
Choline	100–200 mg.
Vitamin C	500–2,000 mg.
Vitamin D	5–20 mcg.***
Vitamin E	50–400 TE.****
Zinc	15–25 mg.
Iron	15–25 mg.
Calcium	800–1,200 mg.
Magnesium	300–800 mg.
Manganese	5–10 mg.
Phosphorus	500–800 mg.
Potassium	500–1,000 mg.
Copper	0.5–2.0 mg.
Molybdenum	10–100 mcg.
Chromium	50–200 mcg.
Selenium	50–200 mcg.
Iodine	100–200 mcg.

*1,000 micrograms = 1 milligram
**Vitamin A activity expressed in Retinol Equivalents (new)
***Micrograms of Cholecalciferol Activity (new)
****Expressed in alpha-tocopherol equivalent

VITAMINS

Vitamin A (Retinol, Carotenoids)

Function: Maintenance of mucous membranes and skin, night vision, bone growth, and reproduction.

Food Sources: Dairy products, dark greens, and yellow fruits.

Toxic Level: 75,000 I.U. (15,000 mcg R.E.)

R.D.A.: 800–1,000 mcg. RE (Retinol Equivalents; the new way of expressing vitamin A activity).

Vitamin D (Cholecalciferol)

Function: Bone formation, calcium and phosphorus metabolism.

Food Sources: Fortified milk, tuna, salmon. Also made by sun's actions in deep skin layers.

Vitamin D (continued)

Toxic Level: 5,000 I.U. in some people.
R.D.A.:   5-10 mcg. (Mcg. of Cholecalciferol Activity).

Vitamin E (Tocopherol)

Function: Many widespread actions in the body. Protects essential fatty acids, acts as an antioxidant. Aids in formation of red blood cells.
Food Sources: Dark green vegetables, wheat germ, whole-grain cereals, vegetable oils.
Toxic Level: Unknown.
R.D.A.:   8-10 T.E. (alpha-tocopherol equivalent).

Vitamin B_1 (Thiamine)

Function: Carbohydrate metabolism, appetite control, nervous system function.
Food Sources: Whole grains, fish, meat, nuts, poultry.
Toxic Level: None.
R.D.A.:   1.0-1.5 mg.

Vitamin B_2 (Riboflavin)

Function: Energy metabolism.
Food Sources: Milk, eggs, whole grains, mushrooms, dried peas and beans.
Toxic Level: None.
R.D.A.:   1.2-1.7 mg.

Vitamin B_3 (Niacin, Niacinamide, Nicotinic Acid)

Function: Works in conjunction with thiamine and riboflavin in energy metabolism.
Food Sources: Poultry, peanuts, whole grains; body can convert the amino acid tryptophan into niacin.
Toxic Level: Low, 3,000 mg. Diabetics and those with peptic ulcers should consult a physician before taking large doses. Flush and itching can occur with niacin and nicotinic acid, but this is harmless.
R.D.A.:   13-19 mg.

Vitamin B₅ (Pantothenic Acid)

Function: Energy metabolism, formation of hormones.

Food Sources: All plants and animals. Poultry, fish, whole grains.

Toxic Level: None.

R.D.A.: None established.

Vitamin B₆ (Pyridoxine, Pyridoxol, Pyridoxamine)

Function: Acts as a coenzyme involved in metabolism.

Food Sources: Whole grains, fish, walnuts, wheat germ.

Toxic Level: None, but supplement less than 300 mg. a day.

R.D.A.: 2.0–2.2 mg.

Vitamin B₁₂ (Cobalamins)

Function: Fat and protein metabolism, production of red blood cells.

Food Sources: Milk, clams, oysters, fish, meat.

Toxic Level: None.

R.D.A.: 3 mcg.

Folic Acid (Folacin)

Function: Co-factor of the B complex. Acts with B₁₂ in synthesizing genetic material, formation of red blood cells.

Food Sources: Raw green vegetables, raw fruit, wheat germ.

Toxic Level: None. Over 1 milligram a day may mask signs of pernicious anemia.

R.D.A.: 400 mcg.

Biotin

Function: Fat and carbohydrate metabolism.

Food Sources: Soybeans, brown rice, dark green vegetables; made in intestinal track by microorganisms. Raw egg prevents biotin absorption.

Toxic Level: None.

R.D.A.: None established.

Choline

Function:	Co-factor of the B vitamins. Metabolism of fats and cholesterol. Possible brain function and memory.
Food Sources:	Lecithin and eggs.
Toxic Level:	None.
R.D.A.:	None established.

Inositol

Function:	Co-factor of the B complex. Total function unknown.
Food Sources:	Wheat germ and lecithin.
Toxic Level:	None.
R.D.A.:	None established.

Para-Amino-Benzoic Acid (PABA)

Function:	Not established. Co-factor of B vitamins. Important in skin and hair growth. Used on the skin, is an excellent sunscreen.
Food Sources:	Whole grains, wheat germ.
Toxic Level:	None.
R.D.A.:	None established.

Vitamin C (Ascorbic Acid)

Function:	Formation of collagen; detoxifies poisons, resists infection, prevents oxidation of other vitamins, blocks formation of cancer-causing nitrosamines.
Food Sources:	Citrus fruits, tomatoes, peppers, melon.
Toxic Level:	None established; diarrhea can occur in high doses.
R.D.A.:	60 mg.

MINERALS

Calcium

Function:	95% used in bones and teeth; nerve function and muscle contraction.
Food Sources:	Milk products, salmon, dark green vegetables.

Calcium (continued)

Toxic Level: None. Avoid megadoses (15,000 mg.), which can cause overload.

R.D.A.:   800–1,200 mg.

Magnesium

Function: Transmission of nerve impulses, pH balance, metabolism, bone structure.

Food Sources: Green vegetables, lemons, grapefruit, apples, whole grains.

Toxic Level: 10 grams magnesium sulphate. Lesser amounts of other forms.

R.D.A.:   300–400 mg.

Phosphorus

Function: Contributes to supportive structure of body (bones and teeth), energy production.

Food Sources: Fish, poultry, meat, eggs.

Toxic Level: None. Excess depletes calcium.

R.D.A.:   800–1,200 mg.

Potassium

Function: Numerous functions, such as muscle contraction, fluid and electrolyte balance, transmission of nerve impulses.

Food Sources: Bananas, citrus fruits, green vegetables.

Toxic Level: None.

R.D.A.:   None established.

Iron

Function: Manufactures hemoglobin; oxygen transportation.

Food Sources: Meats, green leafy vegetables, dried fruits, whole grain cereals.

Toxic Level: 100 mg.

R.D.A.:   10–18 mg.

Copper

Function: Iron and vitamin C utilization; enzyme reactions and the healing process.

Copper (continued)

Food Sources: Highly available in diet (meats, dried beans).
Toxic Level: Up to 10 mg. appears safe but not desirable.
R.D.A.:   None established.

Zinc

Function: Wound healing, metabolism, carbohydrate digestion.
Food Sources: Oysters, egg, whole grains, seafood.
Toxic Level: Unknown.
R.D.A.:   15 mg.

Manganese

Function: Essential part of several enzymes, systems involved in protein and energy metabolism
Food Sources: Fruits, whole grains, green leafy vegetables.
Toxic Level: 40 mg.
R.D.A.:   None established.

Molybdenum

Function: Participates in essential enzyme systems.
Food Sources: Legumes, whole grains, widespread in the diet.
Toxic Level: Possible in excess of 500 mcg.
R.D.A.:   None established .15–.50 mg. recommended.

Chromium

Function: Sugar metabolism; levels decline with age.
Food Sources: Shellfish, whole grains, mushrooms, brewer's yeast.
Toxic Level: Unknown.
R.D.A.:   None; 50–200 mcg. safe level.

Selenium

Function: Acts against oxidative damage to cells. Interacts with vitamin E to assist in utilization.
Food Sources: Wheat germ, seafood, chicken.
Toxic Level: Very toxic; no more than 300 mcg.
R.D.A.:   None established; 50–200 mcg. safe level.

Iodine

Function:	Function of thyroid gland.
Food Sources:	Seafoods, seaweed, iodized salt.
Toxic Level:	Possibly 1,000 mcg.
R.D.A.:	150 mcg.

Questions and Answers

Q: *I have heard that "natural" supplements are better than "synthetic" ones.*
A: When you consider each vitamin separately, there is no difference. Natural vitamins are derived from food, but few vitamin supplements are all natural. Ninety percent of the vitamin pills sold in health-food stores or drugstores contain at least some vitamins from synthetic sources. Those that are all natural are extremely expensive. True natural supplements are yeast, kelp, fish-liver oil, and rose-hip concentrate. Eat food from natural sources, not pills! To supplement means to add something, not to replace it!

Q: *Do manufacturers trick you in advertising when they say "natural"?*
A: Usually. Synthetic vitamin C is called ascorbic acid. Natural vitamin C could be from citrus fruits, rose hips, acerola, or green peppers. On the bottle it might say: "Vitamin C with rose hips." When you look at the list of ingredients it says ascorbic acid. Therefore, the product is synthetic. You could buy rose-hip tablets, which are natural, but I'll bet an orange is cheaper. It's natural, too!

Q: *I eat a lot of junk food. Should I supplement my diet?*
A: It may help, but not much. You're not getting enough natural food to give you good health. It you're going to make a choice, I would rather see you eliminate junk food than use a supplement. Really good health will only occur when you change all of your bad habits for the better.

Q: *Why don't food processors just sell natural foods, like whole-grain breads?*
A: There is more profit in junk! To sell whole grains would cost them more in shipping, storage (refrigeration), loss due to spoilage and, interestingly, loss of sales. Whole grains are more filling, so you eat and buy less! The cost would be higher for whole grains. White bread still sells better because the average person still buys what's cheap, rather than what's nutritious. People buy the cheapest, fluffiest, softest, whitest bread because that's what the advertisers tell them to buy!

Nutritionally aware consumers see the value in paying more for whole-grain products. It's similar to buying gasoline. You can pay now for high-octane gas or you can pay later for repairs.

Q: *What does R.D.A. mean?*
A: The Food and Nutrition Board of the National Academy of Science sets a recommended dietary allowance (R.D.A.) for vitamins and minerals. They do so on the basis of a review of scientific literature about each nutrient. The R.D.A.'s are higher than the amount needed to prevent specific diseases (for example, 10 milligrams of vitamin C prevents scurvy. The RDA is 60 milligrams). Controversy often arises between the board and researchers, as when the board suggested that there was not enough evidence to recommend a dietary change in fat and cholesterol to reduce the risk of heart disease. Doctors across the country blasted the regulators for irresponsible statements and suggested that some of the members had strong ties to the food industry.

Q: *Does the R.D.A. change?*
A: Yes. Since 1943 the list of recommended dietary allowances has been revised about every five years. In the eighth edition (1974) there was no R.D.A. for chromium, selenium, or manganese. The ninth edition (1980) suggests an adequate intake of all three, which supports the theory that nutritional needs and requirements change as more is learned about the importance of nutrients.

Q: *I've heard that B_6 deficiency may be the cause of athero-sclerosis. Should I load up on B_6?*

A: Dr. Kilmer McCully, a professor of pathology at Harvard Medical School, has suggested such a theory. But before you scrap your low-fat diet for B_6 supplements, read on!

Although a lack of B_6 appeared to be the cause, it was pointed out that a diet high in the amino acid methionine caused the deficiency. Foods high in methionine are animal proteins. It appears that people who eat high-animal protein diets get more methionine than B_6, which is needed to break down methionine. Eating fewer animal products reduces the intake of methionine, while a diet high in whole grains will increase the amount of vitamin B_6. In this situation, additional vitamin B_6 is not necessary.

Homocysteine, a very toxic compound, is theorized to cause atherosclerosis. Methionine, an essential amino acid, is broken down to homocysteine, which in the presence of B_6 is converted to a nontoxic compund called cystathionine.

Q: *Is it true that using birth control pills increases the need for vitamins and minerals?*
A: Yes. This is just one example of the things (stress, drugs, etc.) we do to our bodies that may increase our need for nutrients. Dr. Roslyn Alfin-Slater, a nutritionist at UCLA, says women on the pill run the risk of anemia and should increase their intake of vitamin B_2, folic acid, vitamin E, chromium, and zinc. Skin ailments may also occur. The use of the multi-vitamin-mineral supplement we suggest, along with a good diet, should help considerably.

Q: *Isn't my doctor the best source of nutritional information?*
A: Only if he or she developed an interest in nutrition after graduating from medical school and has pursued it! Most doctors learn little or nothing in medical school about preventing ill health with nutrition. If you find a doctor who is really interested in nutrition, you've got the best of both worlds. Such doctors are very interested in prevention and can use nutrition to analyze and correct many medical problems that may occur.

Q: *Don't some very qualified nutritionists suggest that we avoid supplements?*

A: Yes. Dr. Frederick Stare of Harvard and Dr. Roslyn Alfin-Slater of UCLA are both opposed to supplements. In a speech to the Chemistry Department at California State University at Long Beach, Dr. Alfin-Slater stated that vitamin supplements are necessary only "for those who know they don't eat right, those who eat regularly in restaurants, people on reducing diets or recovering from illness or surgery, older people who have a problem of malabsorption, and infants." I don't know what you make of that statement, but to me it includes 99% of the American population! In fairness though, I think she means that if you don't eat a balanced diet of wholesome foods, you may need supplements.

Q: *Can osteoporosis be caused by a calcium deficiency?*
A: Osteoporosis is an abnormal loss of bone matter. The bone becomes porous. It is most common in older people. Fractures, especially hip fractures, can be an indication of the condition. Low calcium consumption is a factor. However, calcium supplements may not prevent the disease since the balance between calcium and phosphorus seems to be important. High-protein diets seem to contribute to calcium loss, as does the high amount of phosphorus found in processed foods and the phosphoric acid in soft drinks.

Q: *Since osteoporosis is becoming so common, especially among women, how might I best prevent it?*
A: Here's some good advice based on the recommendations of Dr. Robert P. Heaney of the American Society for Bone and Mineral Research:

1. *Exercise regularly:* This may be the most important recommendation. Exercise stimulates new bone formation.
2. *Eat a calcium-rich diet:* 1,000 to 1,200 milligrams a day (above the R.D.A. of 800 milligrams), possibly more. Eat low-fat dairy products or supplement for part of this amount if you avoid dairy products.
3. *Avoid excessive intake of vitamins A and D:* They may cause bones to deteriorate if taken in very excessive amounts over a long period of time.

4. *Don't smoke:* Smokers have less bone mass and more fractures than nonsmokers. Smoking clogs small blood vessels that feed the skeleton.

Q: *Is it true that smokers have an increased need for vitamin C?*
A: Yes. This is another example of bad habits causing vitamin deficiencies. Most smokers are deficient in vitamin C. Evidence indicates that the smoker's body may be unable to properly utilize vitamin C. Giving up smoking means eliminating the worst health habit known to humans and is an obviously better solution than vitamin supplements.

Q: *Can nutrition protect you against the flu?*
A: According to Dr. Theodore Cooper, Assistant Secretary of Health during the Carter Administration, the flu vaccine is the "measure of first resort in combating the threat of influenza." Proper nutrition, including adequate vitamin C, may be an important backup to flu vaccine. Dr. Cooper says that he takes fairly large doses of the water-soluble vitamin B complex and vitamin C.

Q: *Will vitamin C prevent the common cold?*
A: Linus Pauling says yes. Others say no. Vitamin C does seem to reduce the symptoms of the cold. For that reason alone, I think it's a better choice than over-the-counter cold remedies that *definitely do not* prevent or cure anything!

Dr. Pauling recommends taking about 500 to 1,000 milligrams at the first sign of a cold and continuing each hour for several hours. If there are still symptoms on the second day, increase the dose to 4 to 10 grams.

Q: *I have heard of taking vitamin E in the form of mixed tocopherols. The salesman at the health-food store says that only the d-alpha tocopherol is active.*
A: D-alpha-tocopherol is the natural form of vitamin E. This is the one case where a natural vitamin is better than a synthetic. Synthetic vitamin E is stated as dl-alpha-tocopherol.

Q: *Don't we need to add salt to our diet for its iodine content?*

A: Adding iodine to salt was a way of mass supplementation for our population to correct an iodine deficiency which occurred in the 1930s in the Plains states because the soil was deficient in iodine. Since too much salt contributes to hypertension, it is suggested you eat seafoods, all high in iodine. If seafood is not part of your diet, kelp tablets or supplements containing iodine are fine. Many vegetables contain iodine *if* the soil they are grown in is not deficient.

Q: *Can some of the nutrients play a role in detoxifying additives and chemical toxins?*
A: Maybe. In a presentation to the hearing of the U.S. Senate Nutrition Subcommittee in 1979, Dr. Arthur Upton, director of the National Cancer Institute, suggested that we eat a diet with adequate amounts of vitamins and minerals. Studies on animals and humans suggest that vitamins A and C have anticancer properties and zinc, selenium, and iron may also play a preventive role.

Dr. Raymond J. Shamberger, a biochemist at the Cleveland Clinic, said that a cancer-causing chemical, maldnaldehyde, which has its highest concentration in animal products, can be thwarted when the diet includes sufficient food high in antioxidants such as vitamins C and E or traces of selenium. Neither doctor suggested supplementing your diet with these antioxidants or mentioned what an "adequate" or "insufficient" amount might be.

Q: *How much vitamin A could be dangerous?*
A: 75,000 I.U. or more is about the toxic level. Dr. Victor Herbert has reported cases of toxicity with doses as low as 25,000 I.U. For maintenance, lower levels than 25,000 I.U. are recommended.

Q: *It seems that a lot of successful athletes take bee pollen. It must have some effect.*
A: A lot of athletes take it and swear by it. Unfortunately, there is not one ounce of evidence that it has any effect on energy. It is high in vitamins and minerals, though. Even Mohammed Ali says he took it, but it must have had a reverse effect in his fight with Holmes! If you have some money to waste, go ahead. It won't hurt you, but don't expect it to vault you into the winner's circle.

Q: *What about vitamin B_{15}?*
A: B_{15} is better known as calcium pangamate. Reports out of Russia imply that B_{15} can enhance performance by increasing our oxygen utilization at the tissue level. It is unclear if these tests were double-blind. Exercise physiologists in America are not too excited about the results. I am unaware of tests done in the United States that support many of the wild claims coming out of Russia.

The good news is that you can get plenty of calcium pangamate from a whole, unprocessed diet. Dr. Richard Passwater, a biochemist and research director of the American Gerentological Research Laboratories, is the strongest proponent of vitamin B_{15}. Although he does not make a specific recommendation for athletes, he states that whole grains, sunflower seeds, and pumpkin seeds are good sources. Rice bran, wheat germ, oat grits, and corn grits are exceptionally high. Once you price B_{15} at the health-food store you will be even more eager to get it from natural sources. Like bee pollen, it's ridiculously overpriced. Get yours naturally from natural carbohydrates.

Q: *I have heard that coffee taken prior to exercise can increase endurance.*
A: Actually, it's the caffeine in the coffee. If there is a positive effect, it is probably true only in distance events. Caffeine increases the free fatty acids in the blood system. This actually spares glycogen so that the runner has more fuel (glycogen) at the end of the race. I doubt that top runners are much improved, since they are already capable of burning fat better. A 3:30 marathoner may be able to knock 10 seconds off that time but that's not going to set any records. For most endurance events, little effect will occur. Don't forget that caffeine causes increased urination, which can result in dehydration. The trade-off may not be worth it.

Q: *It is hard to believe that we don't have a need for more vitamins than we get.*
A: We might! The research isn't conclusive yet. In the meantime, use sound prevention by eating a positive diet supplemented with a reasonable amount of vitamins and minerals. Don't become paranoid about the whole thing!

Q: *Is anemia common in athletes?*
A: More so in women, but I suspect it is high among endurance athletes who expend large amounts of energy. A good example is swimmers who train at 10,000 to 20,000 yards a day. A common cause of anemia is low hemoglobin, which reduces the oxygen-carrying capacity of red blood cells. If you experience a lack of stamina and energy and develop a general feeling of tiredness, you should see a doctor for testing of low hematocrit.

A negative diet, low in iron, can contribute to this type of anemia. Women athletes should supplement their diet with 18 to 30 milligrams of iron. The normal diet does not contain enough iron to meet the needs of female athletes. Joan Ullyot, M.D., a practicing physician in San Francisco, suggests that women take iron if symptoms occur—100 milligrams, three times a day for six weeks. If no change occurs, then have the test. There can be many causes for anemia.

Q: *Is any one vitamin or mineral most important to athletic performance?*
A: No. You're only as good as your weakest link. Since there are well over forty nutrients essential to good health, it's important to eat a well-balanced diet.

Q: *Why not supplement all the nutrients and be sure?*
A: You couldn't get a pill that size into your mouth, and the cost would be prohibitive! Wouldn't eating wholesome food be more enjoyable and cheaper?

Q: *Does vitamin E improve endurance?*
A: I doubt that it has a direct effect. In other words, just adding it to your diet may not improve your endurance. Its effects as an antioxidant may indirectly aid performance if your diet is not already adequate in vitamin E. Athletes who eat a diet deficient in whole grains, legumes, and green leafy vegetables and high in polyunsaturated oils are most likely to experience a deficiency of vitamin E. An improved diet is more essential than supplementing vitamin E, but low-level vitamin E supplements should be of no harm and may contribute to a well-planned nutritional program.

Q: *Can vitamins prevent cancer?*

A: We don't know the answer yet, but preliminary research suggests that they may play a preventive role. Dr. Colin Campbell, professor of chemistry and biochemistry at Cornell University, says a diet high in vitamins A, C, and E and fiber and low in fat is effective in preventing the occurrence of cancer, and may even reverse existing cancer in humans.

6

FOOD ADDITIVES: FRIEND OR FOE?

Let's start this chapter with a test. The following list of ingredients can be found on the label of (a) a nondairy whipped topping (b) motor oil (c) a powdered fruit drink (d) embalming fluid.

Citric acid, gum arabic, natural and artificial cellulose gum, calcium phosphate, sodium citrate, ascorbic acid, hydrogenated vegetable oil, vitamin A, artificial colors, and butylated hydroxytoluene.

The correct answer is "C," but you probably had to guess! Most of us have no idea what's in the food we eat. A recent ad claiming "There's a lot of good chemistry between us" could have been talking about our relationship with our friendly food processor. The use of food additives has become a major infringement on our nutritional environment, and it shows little indication of decline. Few of us are aware of the total impact this can have on our health. Food processors spend millions of dollars every year in their attempt to educate the public about the supposed safety of food additives, while only a few dollars are spent on positive nutritional education.

The average American diet contains large amounts of highly processed foods that are loaded with additives. Everywhere we turn there's advertising and promotion to encourage us to eat more junk food. Cash prizes, toys, vacations, and discounts are all used to entice us to eat a certain cereal or dine out at a fast-food outlet. We've all observed the child in the supermarket screaming for a specific cereal, unable to wait to rip open the box to get the prize. The cereal won't go to waste, though. Mommy paid good money for it, and her offspring is going to eat it, additives, sugar, and all!

Jack LaLanne had a point when he said "eat the carton—throw away the cereal—and play with the toys." At least the carton contains fiber.

The emphasis is on fun, not nutrition. It's *fun* to eat "Mr. Zomm Space Bars," but fresh fruit is a drag! Powdered citrus drinks are fun—they went to the moon—and kids can make it themselves. Who's got time to squeeze oranges?

The end result of all these Madison Avenue gimmicks is that the average adult easily consumes over 3,000 different additives a year in the form of flavorings, colorings, thickeners, emulsifiers, and antioxidants. These are consumed willingly in the quest for fun and convenience, with little thought to the potential health hazards. Millions of dollars in food additives go into processed food every year, bringing the average person's annual consumption to over nine pounds.

The bottom line in the American marketplace is profit. The unpleasant fact is that processed foods and junk foods yield higher profits. That's an economic reality that we must accept. We cannot assume that corporate officers in the food industry spend hours pondering the problem of how to enhance the nutritional status of the world. Their time is spent working to increase the profit margin of every product they produce. The consumer should also accept some of the responsibility for the increased amount of additives found in processed foods. After all, if there was not a consumer out there in the marketplace eagerly buying the product, then the producers would have no market for it.

The Functions
of Food Additives

Let's take a look at the function of some of the most common groups of food additives:

FLAVOR ENHANCERS

Natural ingredients are usually more costly than their artificial counterparts. The flavor enhancer enables the food industry to provide a substitute for a natural ingredient by using a chemical flavor enhancer that accentuates the natural taste. If a label reads "artificial" cherry, it is unlikely that we will find real cherries inside. Instead we will find a chemical substitute that looks, smells, and tastes like cherries and is much more profitable to the manufacturer.

THICKENING AGENTS

Thickening agents give food a rich, thick appearance with good texture and consistency. Unfortunately, they also replace some wholesome ingredients. Ice cream is a good example. Cream and eggs are thickening agents used in natural or homemade ice creams. In an effort to create a cheaper, more profitable product, commercial ice cream manufacturers substitute chemical additives. These thickening agents make ice cream smooth and prevent it from melting and crystallizing. We know it's prudent to avoid highly saturated fats and cholesterol in our diet (from eggs and cream), but it would be nice if we could make that decision ourselves. Many other thickening agents, such as modified starches, make nutritionally inferior products appear more appealing.

ARTIFICIAL COLORS

Artificial colors are the least necessary of all the additives. The function of artificial coloring is to add eye appeal without incurring the cost of using natural foods and colors. Most artificial colors are synthetized from coal and are classified as coal-tar dyes. They are used not only in food but in cosmetics as well.

In 1940 the Food and Drug Administration certified 251,000 pounds of coloring. By 1970 the annual amount had increased to over 3,735,000 pounds! The dyes are used in soft drinks, luncheon meats, cheeses, sausages, hot dogs, pie fillings, baking products, candy, ice cream, puddings, desserts, and a host of other processed foods. Even our pet foods have artificial color.

ANTIOXIDANTS

Chemicals such as BHT (butylated hydroxytoluene) are added to oils to prevent them from becoming rancid. Just about any product that contains oil will have BHT or BHA (butylated hydroxyanisole) listed as an additive on the package. These additives increase shelf life and allow manufacturers to ship larger quantities to supermarkets with little or no spoilage.

VITAMINS AND MINERALS

The addition of vitamins and minerals in the name of "fortification" or "enrichment" enables manufacturers to make nutritional claims for products that are less wholesome than their natural counterparts. We have all seen the television ads for name-brand snacks, which suggest that the products are nutritious because of the added vitamins and minerals. As already shown, white flour is deficient in many nutrients after milling. To enrich white flour does not make it equal to whole-grain flour. The same is true of these snacks. They are made with deficient flour and are filled with sugar and fats, which make no positive contribution to our diet. The list of food processors who make ridiculous claims about their wonderfully "fortified" products is almost endless. Food processors are the worst charlatans in the vitamin-supplement business.

Are Additives Dangerous?

Whether additives are safe is a legitimate question. At this time we can't really be sure that all additives are safe beyond a reasonable doubt. On the other hand, we can't say that they are all dangerous either. As a group, most appear to be safe. Additives can be vitamins, minerals, amino acids, or other nutrients which probably do no harm other than deceiving the public into thinking a product is more nutritious than it really is. However, we cannot assume that because most additives are safe, all are safe. Government regulations have permitted the use of additives which were thought to be safe, only to discover later that these additives were in fact highly toxic. Red No. 2 dye, for example, was finally banned in 1976 because it causes cancer. Red No. 2 once accounted for 35% of all food colorings used in the United States. Over one million pounds of this coal-tar dye were used in 1973. To date, the FDA has banned over twenty-five additives suspected of causing cancer, kidney damage, and other organ damage, after first permitting their use.

Testing for Safety

The FDA has a list of additives called the G.R.A.S. (Generally Recognized As Safe) list. These additives can be used in foods. Prior to 1958, additives were used at the discretion of the manufacturer, and the FDA had to prove an additive dangerous before it could compel the manufacturer to remove it. Since 1958, however, a manufacturer must test the safety of a food additive and submit the results to the FDA for approval.

The major problem with the current system is obtaining objective test results when the company which wants to use a new additive is also doing the testing. In 1976 Dr. Alexander Schmidt, then head of the FDA, said that some research laboratories had deliberately falsified test data on the safety of drugs and chemicals being consumed by the American public. In an article in the *Long Beach Press Telegram* on November 15, 1976, he went on to say, "The nation is going to be in for some rude shocks when the FDA and the National Cancer Institute begin tackling a backlog of 250 compounds for possible cancer and mutagenic hazards."

The Risk Factor

The scientists who represent the food industry point out that even when an additive is labeled as a possible carcinogen (cancer-causing agent), the possibility of getting cancer from its use is so slight as to be insignificant. We are then required to make some decisions based on the risk factor. We assess risk daily in many areas, such as driving our car, playing tackle football, and flying. At some point we must ask, "Is the benefit worth the risk?" With additives that's an important factor to evaluate. As consumers we have to ask ourselves, "If I don't eat product *A* (to avoid additives), what do I lose? Is there an alternative?"

In developing our attitudes toward additives, it's important to look at the specific danger to which we are exposed. We must consider that over twenty-five additives have been declared dangerous and removed from the G.R.A.S. list after they were in use. We must also remember that no one can say with accuracy how many of the additives in use today may prove to be dangerous as the result of future testing. In all probability most additives are safe, but until the results are in, the public is left to play Russian roulette with thousands of unneeded additives.

Additives to Avoid

FOOD COLORINGS

Food colorings serve no nutritional purpose, and some are suspected of causing cancer. It is also suspected that hyperactivity in some children may be related to food colorings. They are the number-one group of food additives to avoid. Let's look at a few:

1. Orange B: Used almost exclusively to color the skin of hot dogs. Chemically related to Red No. 2, which was banned as a carcinogen.
2. Citrus Red No. 2: Colors the skin of oranges and is added to marmalade and candied orange peel.
3. Red No. 40: The substitute for Red No. 2—widely used.

SODIUM NITRITE

Sodium nitrite is primarily used to preserve meats, but manufacturers really like it because it also gives color to the meat. Meats that are loaded with fat, such as hot dogs, sausages, and luncheon meats, have much more eye appeal with that red "meaty" look than the pale, gray look they would have without the addition of sodium nitrite.

Nitrites combine with amines in the body to form nitrosamines. Dr. William Lijinski, a biochemist with Oak Ridge Laboratories, calls nitrosamines the most potent cancer-causing agents yet discovered. In light of current research, the FDA recently lowered the amount of sodium nitrite allowable in bacon and other cured meats. Since sodium nitrite is merely a preservative, it is not absolutely necessary. Refrigeration can reduce the need significantly. Again, however, desire for profit outweighs the possible health hazards. Fortunately, however, the foods that are high in nitrites are also high-fat foods which we should eliminate from our diet for other reasons.

BHT (BUTYLATED HYDROXYTOLUENE)

BHT is a preservative that is totally unnecessary and that is suspected of increasing our risk of cancer. The purpose of BHT is to retard spoilage in foods containing oil. However, many companies seem to do quite well without it. Potato chips are a good example. Although most popular brands contain antioxidants such as BHT, natural chips have been shown to have a long shelf life without these additives. This is probably due to the better handling and packaging of the natural products. Besides, who can't live without potato chips!

The Alternative

Food manufacturers claim that we need additives to feed America. In fact, though, if we eliminated all foods that contain additives it would not have a negative effect on our nutritional state. On the contrary, eliminating most of the foods that contain additives would enhance the nutritional level of the country considerably.

When we avoid additives we also avoid processed foods, junk foods, and "nonfood products," which contain high amounts of nonessential fats, sugar, and calories. The alternative to products that contain food additives is almost always more nutritious.

PRODUCTS THAT CONTAIN ADDITIVES	MORE NUTRITIOUS ALTERNATIVE CHOICES
1. Powdered drinks, canned and bottled sodas	1. Fresh fruit and vegetable juices
2. Sugar-coated breakfast cereals and white breads	2. Additive-free whole-grain cereals and breads without sugar added
3. Instant desserts, puddings, cakes, pies, etc.	3. Fresh fruit, homemade desserts low in fat and sugar
4. T.V. dinners, canned meals, etc.	4. Meals made from natural foods—fresh fish, poultry, some meats, fresh vegetables

Reacting to the Propaganda

We are constantly bombarded with propaganda supporting the use of food additives. Many of the points are not well taken. For example.

1. *Anything can cause cancer in high doses.*
This statement is simply not true. Many chemicals do not cause cancer, even in high doses. Also, it is not clear that there is a minimum level for a carcinogenic agent. A small amount may be just as dangerous as a large amount.

2. *Tests are not economically feasible—they take large sums of money as well as time. To test every chemical for safety is not possible.*
This statement is true, so we had better avoid as many chemicals as possible!

3. *Some additives may be safe alone, but when combined with other chemicals they become toxic.*
True. Some additives are safe alone; it is only in combination with other chemicals that they become toxic. (Nitrites combined with amines in the body to form nitrosamines).

4. *Additives are necessary to feed America.*
We can live very healthfully without additives. Why take the risk when there are so many good alternatives available?

Guide to Reducing Additives in Your Diet

Having determined that additives are a risky business, how can we eliminate them from our diet?

1. *Read labels:* This is the best nutritional education there is. What we can't pronounce we shouldn't be eating! Sugar and caffeine are additives, too. We should avoid them.
2. *Avoid packaged and canned foods:* Use fresh products as much as possible.
3. *Avoid processed snacks:* Chips, cookies, and crackers are not good choices. Reading the label is enough to convince most people.
4. *Avoid junk foods:* Instant pudding, pies, cakes, and candy add calories and unwanted additives, and provide minimal nutrition.

5. *Support companies that use wholesome natural ingredients free of additives:* The cost of these products may be high, but so is their nutritional value. Most of these products taste a lot better as well. If nutritious food becomes profitable, more manufacturers will make it available.

CAFFEINE AND YOUR HEALTH

It is debatable whether caffeine is dangerous. The FDA recently warned pregnant women to limit consumption of coffee and other products that contain caffeine because of the possible connection between caffeine and birth defects.

Caffeine stimulates the central nervous system, which can lead to nervousness, irritability, sleeplessness, anxiety, and heart palpitations. More serious effects, such as peptic ulcer, elevated cholesterol, elevated fat levels, and ventricular fibrillation (irregular heart contractions), have all been associated with high caffeine intake. People with high caffeine intake (more than fifteen cups of coffee a day) may develop "caffeinism," which results in insomnia, fever, and irritability.

At this time no one can say at what level caffeine becomes dangerous, but present knowledge of its effects indicates that we should all reduce our intake. Dr. Alan Goldman of Children's Hospital in Philadelphia says, "We know enough to know it's dangerous."

Most of us know about the caffeine we get from our coffee and tea but are unaware of its presence in other products. Parents often forbid children to drink coffee, because it is "bad for them." The ingredient they are trying to avoid is caffeine. However, these same parents frequently allow their children to drink cola drinks, which all contain caffeine (in fact, if the label says "cola," the FDA requires that caffeine be included in the ingredients). Due to his or her smaller size, a small child consuming three colas a day is actually drinking the equivalent of eight cups of coffee consumed by the larger adult. Parents should be especially concerned about how much caffeine their children consume, since the combination of caffeine with a high sugar intake may cause serious negative consequences. Many American children consume five to ten cola drinks and several candy bars a day—a combination which may permanently damage their health.

Caffeine is found in many products besides coffee and tea. Some products containing caffeine are: candy bars, 25 milligrams; cola drinks (12 ounces), 40 to 72 milligrams; stay-awake pills, 100 milligrams; cocoa (6 ounces), 10 milligrams; coffee (6 ounces), 83 milligrams; tea (6 ounces), 28 to 41 milligrams. Less conspicuous caffeine-containing products are cold remedies such as Excedrin and Anacin, which contain varied amounts of caffeine.

The use of decaffeinated coffee is promoted as an alternative for those who drink coffee. The promoters fail to mention, however, that trichloroethylene, the solvent used to extract the caffeine from the coffee bean, has been found to cause liver cancer in mice. Methylene chloride, which has replaced trichloroethylene, is currently being tested by the National Cancer Institute.

Coffee drinkers need not despair, however. There is one possible alternative that appears to be safe. Some specialty coffee stores sell a decaffeinated coffee obtained by use of the "steam extraction" method, where no solvents are used. There is also a gas extraction method in use in Switzerland. These coffees may be safer, but the price is about $8 a pound, enough to discourage most people. As for tea—linden tea and most Chinese teas are low in caffeine.

SALT AND YOUR HEALTH

We need small amounts of salt in our diet for many important functions: regulation of body fluids, transmission of nerve impulses, heart action, and the metabolism of carbohydrate and protein. The problem is that we get too much salt—and that's definitely not healthy. It is a well-substantiated fact that high-salt diets are strongly associated with high blood pressure (hypertension), which is a major risk factor in the incidence of heart disease. Hypertension is a silent killer with no outward symptoms. Only a blood pressure test, properly interpreted, can identify the disease. A low-salt diet is not only recommended to correct the disease, but is the best preventive measure. It is suggested that we can get along quite well on about two grams of salt a day. Our actual need is probably much less, probably in the neighborhood of 250 to 500 milligrams (1/2 gram). Most people easily consume ten times this amount.

AVOIDING SALT

It is interesting to observe people as they eat. Frequently they will add salt to food *before* even tasting it. Eliminating the salt shaker is a step in the direction of good health. We should not add salt to our food. Those who find food too bland without added salt would be wise to examine the quality and freshness of their food and evaluate preparation methods. Overcooked and over-processed food usually loses much of its natural salt and many of its minerals, which give taste to the food.

The salt shaker is only a part of the problem. It accounts for only 25% of our total salt intake. The rest is found in the bland processed food that's loaded with added salt for taste appeal. Food processors are well aware of how addicted people are to salty food, so they do not hesitate to capitalize on the habit. There is salt added to almost every food we can imagine. Added salt is found in cured meats, bread, soups, canned vegetables, tomato juice, frozen dinners, breakfast cereals, and cakes. They even add salt to ice cream!

It is important to realize that sometimes the label doesn't say "salt." More prestigious names are used, such as sodium nitrite (remember nitrite!), a curing and preservative agent; sodium bicarbonate, a leavening agent; monosodium glutamate, a flavor enhancer; sodium benzoate, a preservative. Look for these on the list of ingredients and avoid them. The ingredients listed on the label start with the predominant ingredient and are listed in descending order of amount. If salt (or sugar, fat, etc.) is listed in the first few ingredients, you know that product has a very high concentration of that ingredient. It is not unusual to find a whole gram of salt per serving in many canned soups.

Dr. Lawrence Powers, in his syndicated column in the *Los Angeles Times*, states, "Take two quick examples of the problem: corn and tomatoes. There is a thousand times more salt in cornflakes than in corn as corn on the cob; and there is an even greater salt jump in catsup from the field tomato." Produce such as fruits, vegetables, and grains all contain sodium, but in a much lower proportion than their processed look-alikes. One potato contains only 5 milligrams of salt while the processed potato chip yields 200 milligrams in only ten chips. A cucumber yields 2 milligrams of salt in seven slices while a dill pickle contains 928 milligrams. As you can see, it's very difficult to avoid salt. If your diet contained only natural products and you avoided all processed foods with added salt, you would still consume an adequate amount of salt to meet your daily requirements. Throw that salt shaker away and start reading labels!

AGRICULTURAL POISONS

Most pesticides used on food crops are used by the large farms involved in monocropping, which sell to our supermarkets. Organic farms and small cooperative farms use few, if any, poisons.

The Environmental Protection Agency has established "limits" of pesticides allowable in food. It is highly questionable whether there really are safe limits. Certainly, the lower the limit, the lower the risk of disease.

Of the 1,500 ingredients found in pesticides, one-third are toxic and one-fourth are known to be carcinogens. Dieldrin, Aldrin, and DDT are three pesticides that were used for many years before being banned in the early 1970s as cancer-causing agents. No one knows how many others still in use have the same effect.

Even if low levels of pesticide actually do not adversely affect our health, we are faced, as a society, with a serious problem. The longer a pesticide is used, the more resistant insects become to it. This resistance is inherited by their offspring, which means that more of the poison must be used to accomplish the purpose.

The five-year report on pesticides published by the National Academy of Science Research Council came to these conclusions (quoted from Knight News Service):

1. Many pesticides destroy not only nuisance organisms but also birds and other creatures that eat insects.
2. High yield "Miracle Crops" have become very susceptible to pests at the very time chemical pesticides are losing their clout.
3. There is evidence that perhaps as many as 100 pesticides are health hazards for man.

ORGANIC PRODUCE

The majority of pesticides and chemical fertilizers are used by the large corporate farms that supply most of the produce we purchase at the market. As a result, many people have turned to health-food stores to purchase supposedly "pesticide free" organically grown produce. While this may give peace of mind to many consumers, the fact is that organically grown food is seldom, if ever, lower in pesticide residue than the less expensive supermarket variety. It's doubtful that the nutritional quality is much better either. Nutritional quality is controlled more by the harvest time, weather, and the plant's genes than by the fact of whether it was grown with organic or chemical fertilizer. In fact, it is more probable that the mineral content will be higher in plants treated with chemical fertilizers than in those treated with organic fertilizers.

Many "reputable" health-food stores are well aware of this fact and therefore do not promote their produce as organic, but simply offer it as a convenience to the shopper.

There are some alternatives we should consider:

1. *Eat more plant foods and less meats:* The concentration of fat-soluble pesticides and other toxic substances goes up as we eat foods higher on the food chain. Animals store pesticides from the plants and water they consume. Humans, in turn, consume the animal and marine life, thus increasing their own concentration of pesticides. Therefore, beef and dairy products are much higher in pesticides than the plant foods that the animals eat. Root vegetables, grains, legumes, fruits, and leafy vegetables have considerably less pesticide concentration than oil, fats, dairy products, meat, fish, and poultry.

2. *Maintain a high nutritional status:* Eating a diet high in vitamins and minerals may block the effect of toxins that get into our bodies through our food chain. Vitamins A, C, and E and the mineral selenium may be most important, but a diet balanced in all the vitamins and minerals is most prudent. For example, Jim Cleveland and T. F. Rees, writing in *Science Magazine,* reported that B vitamins reduce the toxicity of pesticide residues.

3. *Wash all produce:* Always wash fresh fruits and vegetables in a light solution of detergent to get rid of pesticide residues on the surface.

HORMONES, ANTIBIOTICS, AND DRUGS USED ON ANIMALS

A few years ago, the United States General Accounting Office issued a study which found that 14% of the dressed meat and poultry sold in our supermarkets contained illegal residues of chemicals suspected of causing cancer, birth defects, and mutations. Of the 143 drugs and pesticides identified as likely to leave residues in raw meat and poultry, 42 are suspected of causing cancer, 20 may cause birth defects, and 6 show evidence of causing mutations. Obviously, it is not safe to assume that government inspection means that our meats are pure.

To maximize profits by producing high-yield cattle with maximum weight, cattle ranchers resort to drugs. Unfortunately, this may mean that dangerous drug residues remain in the meats we consume.

Diethylstilbestrol (DES) was first approved for livestock use in 1954 by the FDA. DES is a female hormone that was administered to livestock to stimulate weight gain, which means more profit for the livestock owner. By 1972 scientific evidence had shown that DES causes cancer in humans. Because of lengthy court hearings, the final ban on this drug did not occur until seven years later, in 1979. In the meantime, the American people continued to consume DES in their meats. DES is the same drug administered to pregnant women since 1941 to prevent miscarriages. It was banned for that purpose in 1971 when it was found to cause vaginal and cervical cancer in some daughters of women who had taken the drug.

The ill effects of DES were so well known that many foreign countries would not import United States beef because of the DES residue.

Now that this dangerous additive is banned, is everything fine? No! As recently as September 1980, government agencies found that most feed lots were ignoring the ban on DES and in the interest of higher profits were illegally using the drug. From a sampling of 475 feed lots in 23 states, 435,000 DES implants were discovered. The FDA said, "It's very true that we can't prosecute them all, but this is a very serious matter. They showed a wanton disregard for public health." Cattle producers have ignored the scientific evidence. "DES is not a bogeyman," said the head of the California Cattle Feeders Association. "We think it's [the scientific data] a bunch of hogwash." That seems to be the attitude of most food producers when the FDA tries to ban dangerous additives that affect their profits.

It is impossible for you to tell what residues of drugs are present in the meat and poultry you eat, but you can be sure that reduced consumption of animal foods is beneficial. Another alternative is to buy range-fed beef. This beef is leaner and is free from hormones and antibiotics. It is found in many natural-food stores, and it is also quite expensive.

HOW HEALTHY IS YOUR WATER?

No discussion of additives would be complete without mention of our water supply. Anyone who compares municipal water with fresh spring water knows there is a big difference. Spring water tastes better.

The question is: Is municipal water safe? We know it contains pollutants in varying degrees. Nitrate, which is found in many water supplies, can be dangerous to infants under six months of age. Even the chlorine used to kill the bacteria can, under some circumstances, contribute to the formation of carcinogenic chemicals in the water. The relationship of high levels of sodium and cadmium to heart disease have been suspected. Water softeners create an additional problem. They're great for dishes and clothes, but they're too high in sodium (salt) to use in drinking water. While the experts research the safety of municipal water supplies, the public should look for a better alternative.

Bottled water may be the answer, since we don't actually consume much water for drinking. Most of the water we use goes for washing, toilets, lawns, cars, etc. Very little is used for cooking or drinking. Bottled water is usually spring water or purified water with a balance of minerals. It is low in sodium and has a much better taste than most tap water. As a service, most bottled water companies will furnish chemical comparisons between the local water supply and their water. It is important to select a reputable company that is well established in the community. An interesting point in favor of bottled water is that every chemist involved in water analysis with whom I talked drinks bottled water. Do they know something we don't?

Questions and Answers

Q: *What about the major additives in food—sugars?*
A: Sugar is definitely an additive and should be avoided. On labels it can be referred to as sugar, corn syrup, dextrose, or glucose. We consume about 28 billion pounds of sweeteners a year. The higher your sugar intake, the more deficient your diet is likely to be.

Q: *How about sugar substitutes?*
A: These are not a good choice. Cyclamates, the most popular substitute prior to 1970, was banned by the FDA because it

caused bladder cancer in rats. Since it is thirty times sweeter than sugar it was a very economical sweetener for the food processors, who are presently trying to get it back on the market. The current substitute, saccharin, carries a warning that it causes cancer in laboratory animals. That warning doesn't help much because so many people ignore it. Saccharin is likely to be banned in the near future.

Q: *Won't the loss of a sugar substitute hurt diabetics and the obese?*
A: Neither saccharin nor any other substitute plays a significant role in controlling these diseases. They should be controlled by positive, lifelong diet changes! Diabetics and obese people can enjoy small amounts of sweets just like anyone else. It's the excessive intake of sugar that's bad for all of us.

Q: *Why is the ban on additives always related to cancer in rats? Why not humans?*
A: That's always been the big joke (it's Johnny Carson's favorite), and you can bet the food processors promote that feeling. It's assumed that if a substance causes cancer in rats it doesn't necessarily mean it can cause it in humans. In the case of saccharin, the promoters suggested that a person would have to drink 1,000 soft drinks to get the same amount that caused cancer in the test rats. This is not true. If rats get cancer, there's a *good* chance humans will, but no one can run such tests on humans. Would you be a volunteer? You don't have to drink 1,000 sodas a day. If your intake is average—498 soft drinks a year containing saccharin—that could be enough. High doses are used by cancer researchers for good reasons. They use a small number of animals (because of cost), the animals have a fast rate of metabolism and excretion (it takes 20 to 30 years for cancer to show up in humans), and the animals have a short life span (rodents live only two years). Researchers know that if high doses cause cancer, low doses would cause it in humans as well, although less frequently.

Q: *Are additives in our food the leading cause of cancer from food?*
A: Not according to present knowledge. A high-fat diet, excessive polyunsaturated fats, excess calories (obesity), low fiber, and alcohol all seem to be bigger risk factors at this time. Later

research may change this view, so I suggest you ask this question: "Do I need these additive-rich foods to be healthy?" Reducing your intake of nonessential foods high in additives would be a prudent step toward better health. Removing additive-rich foods also reduces high-fat, low-fiber, and high-calorie foods as well.

Q: *I have heard that some chemicals found naturally in food are toxic and could cause cancer. Why worry about additives?*
A: Aflatoxin, a carcinogen produced by mold, is sometimes found in peanuts. Potatoes and spinach contain a natural chemical that denies calcium to bones. There are traces of cancer-causing chemicals in cabbage, lettuce, and other greens. Neither the environment nor the food supply can be totally risk-free, although the reduction of natural toxins can be accomplished by better storage and production. But this fact should not stop us from controlling *unnecessary* chemicals added to the food and environment. It was not until the addition of synthetic chemicals became prevalent that the national increase in cancer occurred. Dr. Arthur Upton, director of the National Cancer Institute, put it more bluntly: "The soundest principle is, thou shalt not add a carcinogen to the nation's food supply."

Q: *I've heard that hyperactivity may be related to additives children eat in processed foods.*
A: Dr. Benjamin Feingold, a San Francisco pediatrician, was the first to suggest this relationship. The main additives to avoid seem to be the flavorings and colorings. In a Santa Cruz, California school, 16 of 25 hyperactive children showed definite improvement when placed on a diet free of all artificial flavors and colors. Overactivity can also lead to impaired attention span and learning difficulties. Although there are still questions about the long-range effects of Dr. Feingold's diet, there is no argument that it's an improvement. When you couple the additives, sugar, and caffeine found in the typical breakfast of most children, it's no wonder that so many are hyperactive!

Q: *What about nondairy cream substitutes for coffee?*
A: Terrible! Read the labels. They're usually hydrogenated fats and chemicals. Use skim milk or even cream, but consider your total fat intake.

Q: *I'm concerned about the hormones and stimulants in beef. We consume a lot in our family.*
A: Putting it in perspective, I would recommend eating less beef because of its high fat content. Fat is a more important factor in heart disease, cancer, and possibly other diseases than are growth stimulants and hormones in meat. By reducing your beef intake, you accomplish both goals. If hormones are found later to be a major contributor to disease, then you're safe.

Q: *So much seems to cause cancer today that it hardly seems worth the effort to do anything to avoid it.*
A: This should alert you to how much our environment has changed as we introduce new chemicals into our ecosystems. We should all be aware of the potential dangers of adding chemicals to the environment. Eventually, they can have a direct effect on our health when they enter our bodies through water, food, and air. Put in perspective, smoking and exposure to chemicals such as asbestos are more significant in their relationship to cancer, but avoiding any suspected carcinogens, such as some food additives, is a prudent practice. Fortunately, most of the chemicals related to cancer can be avoided without any hardship, if we will just make the effort. Make the obvious changes for your own personal health, and support groups that want to protect the environment.

Q: *Why don't manufacturers eliminate all the additives and produce natural, wholesome food?*
A: This may hurt, but here it goes! To use all natural ingredients would increase the cost of making the product, while shipping problems, cold storage, and increased spoilage would increase the distribution costs. The end result is that the public would get an excellent product, but the cost would be much higher. The manufacturers know that the public is almost totally ignorant of good nutrition, and their surveys prove that people will buy white breat at 75 cents a loaf rather than nine-grain stone-ground whole wheat bread at $1.50. People who are nutritionally aware realize the long-term advantage of whole grains and pay the extra cost, but most people don't. When a significant portion of our population shifts to buying nutritious, rather than low-cost,

products, the manufacturers will improve their products to meet the demand of the majority. If the consumers do not wake up to the facts—the need for more self-education on nutrition and the dangers of junk, low-quality, and inexpensive-to-produce foods (those highly promoted by the food industry because they yield the highest profits)—then we can expect they will continue to offer us low-quality foods.

Q: *I understand that nitrates, which form nitrosamines, are found naturally in vegetables. Why should I worry about nitrates and nitrites added to processed meats?*
A: Vegetables do contain nitrates, but they also contain vitamins. Both vitamins C and E have been shown experimentally to block the formation of nitrosamines.

7
WEIGHT CONTROL: HOW TO KEEP FAT OFF PERMANENTLY

Why, if fad diets are so successful, is there always a new one in style? The reason is simple. People want to believe that there is a special food or a special diet that will let them lose weight without giving up all of their bad habits. It seems that the stranger the diet, the more popular it becomes. Even as I write this chapter, a book on a new fad diet (named for an upper-class city) is hitting the best-seller list. It's unsound, unhealthy, and totally inadequate for healthy weight loss. Yet people will buy the book and go on the diet, envisioning some personal association with the "Beautiful People" of the title community. In the end, failure (if not malnutrition) will surely occur. Most of the popular books on weight control are worthless. The fact that fat people have read all of them should be proof enough. If they worked, the first book would do the trick and its readers wouldn't need to buy any others. The mistake people make is looking for quick results. If you want quick results, then you haven't really committed yourself to trimming down.

Simply put, successful weight control will only occur when you are motivated to change your life-style. Your life-style got you fat, so it's going to take a change in that life-style, especially in your attitude toward food and possibly more importantly toward exercise, to get you thin. They really go hand-in-hand in a practical weight-control program.

Do Calories Count?

Yes, the rule is still true: If you take in more calories than you burn you will gain weight, and if you burn more calories than you take in you will lose weight. Seems simple, doesn't it? Well, it's not quite that simple. Recent research suggests that there may be more to it than just calories in and calories out.

Low-Calorie Diets Make You Fat

You have to burn 3,500 calories to burn one pound of fat; so it seems logical that if you require 2,000 calories to maintain your weight, a low-calorie diet of 500 calories a day should give you a daily loss of 1,500 calories. That translates into 10,500 calories or a weight loss of 3 pounds a week. Sounds typical, doesn't it? After starving on this meager diet for about one month, you'll find that you have lost over 12 pounds. That's right, over 12 pounds! It might be closer to 20 pounds. The additional loss, besides the fat, comes from water and protein; but we'll discuss that later. Now that you've lost your 20 pounds, you're ready to eat normally again. Here's where the problem starts.

You have probably heard about "set point" or "fat point" theory. Basically it says that the body seeks to maintain its level of fat within a narrow range. It is theorized that when you reduce your calorie intake too much, the body responds by increasing your appetite and/or reducing your level of activity to conserve fat. If this doesn't work the body decreases the metabolism, which means you require fewer calories. When you start to eat normally again, but still eat fewer than your required 2,000 calories, you may see the weight creep back. What's happened? The body has a new "set point." It has reduced its metabolism because you tricked it when you went on the low-calorie diet. It's conserving its energy. Thus you now require less than 2,000 calories to maintain weight. In practice this may explain why dieters always complain that they're eating less but can't seem to lose weight as easily.

A second problem with low-calorie diets is that the weight that is lost is not all fat. Actually, water accounts for a large part of the loss and so does protein. That protein comes from your muscle tissue, which is not only unhealthy but also has adverse effects on your body contour. Actually, dieters lose protein and "gain fat." Remember, the body needs to conserve its energy (fat) if you're going to starve it! Your weight may come down, but that doesn't mean the loss is all fat.

Why Fat People Have Difficulty Losing Fat

Our bodies have a wonderful way of adapting to our environments. When we train our bodies through exercise, they adapt to that stress by becoming more efficient. Since muscles are always involved in exercise, they tend to store more fuel. The carbohydrate we eat as food is converted to glucose and travels through the blood. It is stored as glycogen in muscle tissues and in the liver. If the muscles need fuel, they can convert this glycogen back to glucose. An exercised body stores more glycogen in the muscle so it will be available for use when needed. A well-trained body also learns to utilize more fat as a fuel source, conserving the limited stores of glucose in the muscle. This is an important reason why marathon runners can go so long without exhaustion. Their bodies learn to draw more on the fat tank, which has an unlimited supply of fuel, and less on the glucose tank, which is limited.

The exercised individual has a much better chance of staying slim. When he or she eats, the muscles readily take up the glucose and store it for future energy expenditure. It's as if the body is programmed for exercise, so it stores fuel for that purpose. If this glucose were not needed, it would be stored as fat. For the overly fat individual with flabby untrained muscles, the situation is much different. Since the muscles are not called upon for much work, they tend not to store as much glucose. When glucose is traveling in the blood it only has three choices: it can be used as fuel, stored in muscles or liver as glycogen to be used as a source of energy, or stored in fat cells where it is changed to body fat. When the blood glucose level is high, insulin stimulates the muscles to pick up the glucose. The muscles of fat people are resistive to this, so the glucose is routed to the area of least resistance, the fat cells. This tends to make the fat person easily susceptible to getting fatter.

Sedentary fat persons are high carbohydrate burners, because they are in such poor condition. Every time they move they demand large amounts of oxygen. If they participate in high-intensity exercises they force their bodies to burn glucose (carbohydrates), not fat! Because they burn large amounts of glucose, they usually become hungry after exercise, stimulating them to eat and causing more glucose to be stored in the fat cells. It's highly probable that fat people who don't exercise tend to store more of the calories they eat as fat.

Calories do count, but it's the quality of the calories you eat and the amount you're able to metabolize that is important to weight control. Let's look at how exercise can help you increase your metabolism and get you on the road to a healthier and more enjoyable weight-control program.

The Role of Exercise in Weight Control

Our tendency is to look at the problem of weight control as a strictly dietary problem. Ninety percent of our effort is involved with reducing the number of calories we eat, while little attention is paid to the importance of exercise in stimulating that sluggish metabolism and helping you burn more calories. So-called experts sometimes point out that we would have to exercise continuously for five hours to burn off one pound of fat—an unreasonable expectation. Walking one hour a day, they advise, will burn only 300 calories and that can be accomplished more successfully by calorie restriction. The error in this logic is basic. They are saying that if we don't experience immediate results it's not worth the effort. Let's forget for a moment the obvious benefits derived from a physical fitness program and concentrate on its contribution to weight control. Walking for an entire hour to burn only 300 calories hardly seems worth the effort—until we look at the long-range effects. Since 3,500 calories is equal to one pound, every time we burn off (through exercise) 3,500 calories we lose one pound of fat, or we can eat 3,500 additional calories without gaining that pound. Let's assume we balance our calorie intake at the point where we don't gain or lose weight. At this point we take up walking one hour a day and burn 300 calories. If we kept this program up for one year, we would burn 109,500 calories. We would have lost 31 pounds of fat! Those who are in a hurry, like most Americans, would notice that after five days their weight had not dropped much. Even after twelve days it's only down one pound. This causes most people to decide that it's not worth the effort. They quit before they ever experience the positive long-range effects!

The ideal weight-control plan combines a low-calorie diet with exercise. In the situation described above, if we stick with the exercise program and walk off 300 calories a day, at the same time reducing our diet by 300 calories, we would double our long-range loss. At the end of a year the weight loss would be 62 pounds, a little over one pound a week. As fitness levels are reached, activities like running, jogging, cycling, and swimming, which burn even greater amounts of calories, can be undertaken. Take long distance running as an extreme example. People watch these runners go by with sweat rolling down their lean and trim bodies and wonder, "Why can't I be naturally trim like them?" Anyone can—if they will. We can do anything we want, if we'll just do it! That distance runner probably burns 1,000 calories an hour. That's two pounds of fat a week or 104 pounds a year! Runners obviously don't lose that amount. The exercise simply allows them to eat more food and still stay lean and trim. People who exercise aerobically on a regular basis seldom encounter a weight problem because their bodies fully utilize the calories they eat.

ESTIMATED CALORIES BURNED PER MINUTE
DURING SELECTED ACTIVITIES*

ACTIVITY	BODY WEIGHT					
	100	125	150	175	200	225
Basketball						
(Moderate)	5	6	7	8	10	11
(Competitive)	6	8	10	12	14	15
Cycling						
6 MPH	3	4	5	6	7	8
13 MPH	7	9	10	12	15	16
Hiking	5	6	7	8	9	10
Jumping Rope (Moderate)	6	8	9	11	12	13
Mountain Climbing	7	8	10	12	14	15
Rowing Machine	9	11	14	16	18	20
Running 5 min. mile	13	16	20	23	27	29
Running 7 min. mile	10	13	16	19	21	23
Running 8 min. mile	9	12	14	17	19	21
Running 11 min. mile	7	9	11	13	15	16
Running in place (high)	16	20	24	28	32	35
Swimming (25 yds. 1 min.)	3	4	5	5	7	8
Swimming (50 yds. 1 min.)	7	9	11	13	15	17
Walking (2.0 mph)	2	3	4	5	6	7
Walking (4.5 mph)	4	6	7	8	9	10

*Multiply calories times minutes of exercise (Walking 4.5 mph for 60 min., weight 200 = 9 × 60 = 540 Calories)

SLOW DOWN TO LOSE WEIGHT

The good news for those of you who shudder at the thought of exercise is that slow exercise, like walking, is just as good as intense exercise, like running, for burning calories. The basic misconception about exercise is that you must work out vigorously to lose weight. That's just not true! You burn about the same number of calories whether you walk or run three miles. It doesn't sound right, does it? The difference is the time it takes you, not how fast you go. Let's assume you burn 7 calories a minute and it takes you 60 minutes to walk 3 miles. That's 420 calories burned. If you ran that three miles you might burn 14 calories a minute, but it will only take you 30 minutes, so you still burn 420 calories. Another positive principle of low-intensity exercise is that you burn more fat than carbohydrate. How important this is to actual fat loss is still unclear, but it does seem that fat loss increases with low-intensity exercise. Low intensity can vary with the individual; if you're in better condition, a faster pace may still be low intensity. A trained runner can run for a long time at a 7-minute-per-mile pace and still be at low intensity, while a sedentary individual may find a fast-paced walk too intense. It's all controlled by your ability to utilize oxygen. For weight control the rule of thumb is to maintain an intensity that does not cause you to strain for oxygen (such as in a sprint). This would indicate that the intensity is not too high. If you're sedentary and start a walking program for weight control, you will find your ability to tolerate a higher intensity with less stress will occur. This indicates that your condition has improved, which means you can go faster for longer periods of time. That translates into a higher metabolism and more fat loss. The key is low intensity for a longer duration.

REPLACE FAT WITH MUSCLE
TO BURN MORE CALORIES

Most fat people eat less or the same as lean people yet they still gain weight. Why? It may have to do with the ratio of muscle tissue to fat tissue. Your muscle tissue burns about 90% of the calories you consume, so it seems logical that if you have more muscle mass you require more calories. It you're fat, then your ratio goes the other way. Let's say you weigh 200 pounds with 40% fat. That means your muscle or lean body weight is only 120 pounds. Since your muscles burn most of your calories, then you actually only need the calories of a person who weighs about 140 pounds. Fat people burn fewer calories per pound of total body weight. The best way to reduce fat without losing muscle tissue is with exercise. As your percentage of body fat goes down the exercise stimulates muscle growth, which burns more calories. This explains why lean people appear to be able to eat more food. Using our example above, if this person had only 15% body fat instead of 40% fat, his or her lean body weight would be 170 pounds. The total body weight of both is 200 pounds, but the one with the lower body fat has more muscle mass and can, therefore, eat more calories and not gain weight.

You will remember that people who use very restricted diets without exercise actually gain fat and lose muscle mass. If you drop 30 pounds through dieting alone a lot of the weight loss will be from muscle tissue, not fat. So even though your total weight may be lower, you'll still be fat! We see this all the time in sedentary people as they age. Although their total weight does not change from age 25 to age 40, they still look fat. They have lost muscle tissue and gained fat tissue.

ARE YOU OVERWEIGHT OR JUST FLABBY?

Weight charts based on height are not very reliable guides. At best, they are just averages of what other people weigh, rather than ideal weights for specific individuals. Our ideal weight should reflect a lean body with a small amount of fat. Looking in the mirror usually tells the tale. If the body we see in the mirror is not visually appealing, then it is probably too fat! Another simple test is to pinch the skin at the tricep muscle, which is located in back of the upper arm, with the forefinger and thumb. If the thickness of the skin is one-half inch or more, too much fat is being carried. Most of us can tell if we are fat or not, but sometimes we do the wrong thing about it. People who are a bit flabby and lack muscle tone may benefit more from an exercise program than from weight loss. Many young women who are obsessed with being skinny and diet constantly are really on the wrong track. Their problem isn't pounds, it's firmness. One woman could easily weigh 120 pounds and look great, while a friend of the same height could weigh only 110 pounds and look fat. The best way to determine your ideal weight is by body fat measurements.

BODY FAT: HOW TO DETERMINE YOUR IDEAL WEIGHT

People who say they want to lose weight really mean that they want to lose fat. Before starting a weight-loss plan, we should understand more about body fat. On the average, males should have a body-fat range between 12% and 15% and women between 18% and 22%. The range of fat is higher for women than for men because women carry more fat than men for the protection of the uterus and because of hormone variations. Some studies on women athletes have indicated that current ideal listings may be high. As more women take up athletic and fitness programs, the ideal body-fat range may drop. Athletes and fitness enthusiasts usually have lower percentages of fat than the ranges given. Highly trained endurance athletes are sometimes 5% body fat and less.

Once we know the appropriate percentage of body fat, we can determine a person's ideal weight. If a young woman weighs 120 pounds and has a body fat of 30%, we know she's too fat. Her ideal body fat should be between 18% and 22%. At 30% body fat she is carrying 36 pounds of fat ($120 \times 30\% = 36$ lbs.). What's left is her lean body weight, in this case 84 pounds ($120 - 36 = 84$ lbs.). To determine her ideal weight at 18% fat we divide her lean body weight by 0.82 ($100 - 18 = 0.82$); this gives an ideal weight of 102 pounds.

We can determine the percentage of body fat in two ways. The first is the skin-fold measurement using skin calipers. In this method a technician takes several skin-thickness measurements on the body. Applying a formula, he or she can estimate the percentage of body fat.

The second method is much simpler, but less readily available. Since fat floats, an accurate measure of lean body weight and a determination of the percentage of body fat can be made by underwater weighing. Local colleges, the YMCA, etc. are the best places to inquire about this technique. If they don't do it, they will probably know someone who can.

GOOD EXERCISES FOR WEIGHT CONTROL

The best exercises for burning calories are aerobic exercises. Aerobic means "with oxygen." These exercises stimulate and strengthen the heart and lungs. The following are good aerobic exercises:

jogging	stationary cycling	swimming
cycling	running in place	stair climbing
walking	rope jumping	running

Since the purpose of this discussion is weight control, it is important to remember the basic principle: low intensity/high duration. Those who choose to jog, for example, should start off slowly and go farther rather than running fast for a short distance. This causes fat calories to burn. As condition and oxygen utilization improve the runner will be able to go faster and farther, while still burning fat. As our condition improves, so does our ability to metabolize fat.

EXERCISES TO AVOID

All exercise burns calories, but at different levels. Strength exercises, such as weight training, or short intermittent activities, such as tennis, racketball, football, etc., may not be the best activities for weight loss. They burn considerably fewer calories than continuous movement exercises like jogging, and they can take much more time. They are very worthwhile activities to include in a total fitness program, but if weight loss is your main goal and your time is valuable I would suggest you spend it on the activities that will burn the most calories.

Weights are a good example. You could easily spend an hour lifting weights and burn only 200 calories. The reason for this is because your actual "lifting" time may be only 15 minutes; the rest of the time is spent adjusting the weights, talking, and resting. You could have walked for that hour and burned twice that many calories with less effort.

We should exercise to attain between 65% and 75% of our maximum heart rate. A simple rule of thumb for this measurement is to subtract your age from 220 and multiply that figure by 65% and 75%. For a woman 30 years of age that would be a range of 123–142 beats per minute. (220 − 30 = 190 M.H.R. × 65% and 75% = 123–142 training rate)

HOW TO START EXERCISING
FOR WEIGHT CONTROL

Since the amount of oxygen used gives the best indication of how strenuous an activity is, we should monitor our heart rate to ensure that we don't overexert. Someone badly out of condition may find that just jogging slowly for one block puts the pulse rate over the training rate. That person should start the exercise program by walking. Remember, if breathing is too heavy, too many carbohydrates are being burned. We want to burn fat! A highly conditioned individual with the same rate as yours may jog six miles and never hit the training maximum.

As body condition improves, the stress of each workout lessens, and we see our work output increase, while the heart rate stays the same. Our body also will begin to utilize oxygen better, which not only burns more calories, but burns *fat*!

FREQUENCY—DURATION—INTENSITY

As our condition improves, we can raise the training rate above 75%. Athletes in top condition usually train at 85% of maximum, but their goal is optimum fitness rather than just weight control.

I would suggest that you exercise daily at first. This will get that metabolism perked up and alert your body to the new you! As your condition improves, a *minimum* of four days a week at 75% of your maximum rate for 30 minutes of sustained activity will develop an adequate level of cardiovascular fitness and free you from dieting forever.

How the Food You Eat
Affects Your Weight

We mentioned earlier that calories do count, but that doesn't mean you have to count them. Even if you did count calories you would probably be wrong. You could be off by a few hundred calories just by making a few incorrect estimates of the calorie content of each food. Calories are great for making comparisons or explaining a principle of weight loss, but in practical application they are not much help, and few people will count them anyway.

The food you eat is important, and you do have to reduce calories; but that can be accomplished by reducing the foods that contribute most to your excess calorie intake.

Eating Fewer Calories
Without Eating Less Food

It has always been assumed that to reduce calories you must eat less food. That is not totally true. The key to eating fewer calories is to reduce your intake of low-density food and increase your intake of high-density food. From a calorie standpoint, low-density foods contain too many calories for the amount of food you actually eat. Generally these foods are high in fat and/or sugar. In selecting a serving of meat, for example, if you ate 3½ ounces of choice top sirloin, which is high in fat, you would consume about 400 calories. Selecting 3½ ounces of a leaner cut, such as flank steak which is low in fat, you would consume about 200 calories. You reduce your calorie intake but still eat the same amount of food.

High-density foods are usually lower in calories. The lean cut of meat had fewer calories because there was less fat. The higher-density foods are usually naturally occurring complex carbohydrates. Their high fiber content tends to fill you up and has many health advantages that I described earlier in the book. With the exception of a few items, such as avocados, nuts, and legumes, you can eat a considerable amount of these nutritious carbohydrates and still maintain a low-calorie diet.

138

By cutting your servings of high-fat animal foods and eating more high-density complex carbohydrates you can easily reduce your total calorie intake by 500 calories without starving. In fact, Dr. David Costill, director of the Human Performance Laboratory, Ball State University, has suggested that a diet composed of 70% complex carbohydrates in conjunction with an exercise program may be the best balance for weight loss. Remember, we don't want that calorie intake to get too low, or it may reduce our metabolic rate even lower.

FATS: A SOURCE
OF TOO MANY CALORIES

By now it should be obvious that carbohydrates aren't the cause of obesity. All foods have calories. It is simply eating too much food that causes overweight. Since we eat a variety of foods, the secret is to eat more of the foods with low calorie counts. Fat has a higher concentration of calories gram for gram than does protein or carbohydrate.

1 GRAM OF:

Fat   = 9 calories
Protein   = 4 calories
Carbohydrate   = 4 calories

Visually, a regular cube of margarine is rather small, but it contains over 1,000 calories. By adding it to sandwiches, sauces, and other cooking, it is easy to add 500 calories to our diet and never notice it. In contrast, a head of lettuce has only 30 calories. Visualize the difference. To consume 500 calories, less than the amount of calories in one-half cube of margarine, we would have to eat 16 heads of lettuce!

Learning to identify high-fat foods and avoid them allows us to eliminate unwanted calories *without* reducing the quantity of food we eat. That's right! It isn't necessary to starve to lose weight. Here are some general rules:

1. *Most animal products are high in fat:* Choose the ones with the fat removed or reduced (for example, skim milk).
2. *Most processed foods have added fat:* Convert those grams to calories to identify them.
3. *All plant foods are essentially fat-free or very low in fat:* Until you add sauces or dressing—which average about 100 calories a tablespoon!

Let's look at a few examples of foods we eat that contain fat. You will notice that if you choose the first selection you will eat the same amount of food, but considerably fewer calories, than if you choose the second selection:

FIRST SELECTION	SECOND SELECTION
• 8 oz. skim milk = 90 calories	• 8 oz. whole milk = 160 calories
• 1 cup "uncreamed" cottage cheese = 170 calories	• 1 cup "creamed" cottage cheese = 260 calories
• 3 oz. lean meat = 180 calories	• 3 oz. choice meat = 300 calories
• 2 slices chicken breast (no skin) = 83 calories	• Chicken wing (fried) = 151 calories
• 1 can tuna (packed in water) = 251 calories	• 1 can Tuna (packed in oil) = 570 calories
• Baked potato (no butter) = 100 calories	• Baked potato (2 t. butter, 2 t. sour cream) = 280 calories
• Mixed green salad = 50 calories	• Mixed green salad (4 t. dressing) = 230 calories
• 1 box Popcorn (plain) = 25 calories	• 1 box Popcorn (2 t. butter) = 115 calories

The general rule is: The less fat we eat the more food we can eat!

If, on Monday, we were to eat everything in the first selection, our total calorie intake would be 949. On Tuesday, if we ate all the foods in the second selection, we would be consuming 2,066 calories. We would be eating over twice as many calories but not one ounce more food! Fats are the biggest enemy of weight control. Certainly, without *any* fat, food would be less appetizing, but it is really easy to reduce fat calories simply by selecting nonfat and low-fat products and by using less dressing, sauces, creams, butter, and oils.

HOW REFINED SUGAR MAKES YOU FAT

Sugar is classified as a carbohydrate, which means it yields four calories per gram—the same number as protein, but less than half the calories of fat. We could interpret this to mean that sugar is fine in a weight-loss program, but it is not! Refined sugar is nutrient-free. It gives us calories, but no vitamins, minerals, or other nutrients.

Those sneaky little sugar calories aren't just found in sweets, where we expect them. Sugar is added to almost every processed or canned food to replace the natural flavor lost by over-processing. Reading the labels tells us that there is sugar added to mayonnaise, catsup, salad dressing, soup, bread, rolls, peanut butter, luncheon meats, almost anything we can name. If we walked through the supermarket and picked up only the pro-cessed foods without added sugar, our shopping cart wouldn't be very full.

What's wrong with a little sugar? It adds more than a few calories and no nutrients! Canned fruits are a perfect example. One can of pears with sugar contain 113 calories more than pears packed in water. We get the same amount of pears, but the sugar contributes a lot of empty calories. If we chose to eat pears canned in syrup instead of water-packed pears for breakfast every morning for one year, we would have consumed 41,245 empty calories from sugar. That is almost 12 pounds of body weight. The sad fact is, we ate exactly the same amount of pears; only the sugar made the difference. The best choice is to avoid the processed foods altogether and to select a fresh pear at 80 calories. It tastes good, contains fiber, and has more nutrients. Best of all, it's lower in calories.

An important fact to remember about refined sugar is that in processed foods, especially sweets, refined sugar is usually associated with fats. We usually think of pastry, candy, pie, and cake as "sweets," but we forget that sometimes as many as half the calories in these products are fat. At 9 calories per gram of fat, it's easy to see how a small candy bar can contain 250 calories.

Let's look at some additional comparisons to see how hidden fats and refined sugar can increase our calorie intake:

- 1 ounce of fudge is the same as eating 1 large banana: 115 calories
- Eating 6 fresh apples is the same as eating 1 piece of apple pie: 300 calories
- Eating 7 boxes of plain popcorn is the same as eating 1 ounce of peanuts: 180 calories
- Eating 2 oranges is the same as drinking 1 soft drink: 100 calories
- Eating 1 cantaloupe is the same as eating 10 jelly beans: 104 calories

You don't have to eliminate any of these high-calorie products from your diet, but you do have to recognize their contribution to increasing your total calorie intake. Fill up on the nutritious complex carbohydrates first, and use the sweets for treats on special occasions.

LIMITING CALORIES IN YOUR DIET

1. Pay special attention to the "Selection to Limit" list in the chapter on Food Selection.
2. Reduce your intake of:
   Fats
   Refined sugars
   Refined flour products
   Added salt
3. Select high-density foods from:
   Vegetables
   Fruits
   Whole grains
   Legumes
4. Reduce your intake of: And substitute:
   Fatty meats   Lean fish
   High fat dairy products   Chicken and turkey breasts
                                 Nonfat dairy products
5. Exercise aerobically on a regular basis.

SUGGESTIONS FOR REDUCING CALORIES—NOT FOOD

- Read labels: Identify products with excess fat, sugar, refined flour, and salt.
- Convert: Convert grams to percentage of calories to identify the percentages of nutrients you're eating.
- Eat smaller portions: Limit animal and dairy products.
- Eat more: Mixed salads, vegetables, whole fruits, whole grains.
- Limit desserts and sweets: Limit your intake of sweets. No one needs sweets every day!
- Pay Back: If too many calories are eaten, they can be "paid back" with exercise or by eliminating foods at other meals. (For example, if an extra 200 calories are eaten, exercise to lose an additional 200 calories.)
- Limit dressing, sauces, etc: Cut down the amount used or substitute lemon, vinegar, wine, or other low-calorie products. Use more herbs and spices.
- Eat more small meals: Spread your eating pattern among six small meals. This can be done by snacking on fruit, crackers, or mixed vegetables between meals. Save part of a meal to eat an hour or two later. This technique will stabilize your blood sugar, which will reduce your appetite for more food.
- Weigh yourself regularly: Weight loss should be about one pound a week. If not, reduce total calories and/or exercise more.

TIPS FOR EATING OUT

- Request that all butter and sauces be served on the side—this allows total control over how much you use.
- Split dinners, sandwiches, etc.
- Ask for cooked vegetables without butter added.
- Order a la carte.
- Order hors d'oeuvres instead of a full dinner.
- Fill up on the low-calorie foods first.
- Select restaurants with salad bars (easy on the dressing).
- Order baked potatoes (butter on the side, of course).
- Eat cereal rather than eggs, bacon, and hash browns.
- Order one egg instead of an omelette.
- Avoid fried foods (either deep-fried or pan-fried).

PREPARING FOODS AT HOME

- Broil or roast—do not fry or deep fry.
- Steam vegetables.
- Cook without added butter, margarine, and oils.
- Do not add salt to anything.
- Trim fat from meats.
- Eat open-faced sandwiches (using 1 slice of bread instead of 2).
- Put more lettuce, tomatoes, etc. in sandwiches—less tuna, meat, chicken, etc.
- Mix more vegetables and legumes into casseroles than meat or cheese.

SHOPPING

Avoid:
- Processed and packaged foods
- Canned foods
- Frozen foods (second choice)
- High-fat foods

Include:
- Fresh produce and grains
- Fresh meat, fish, poultry
- Nonfat dairy products.

How Fast Should You Lose Weight?

Americans are always in a hurry. We want and expect immediate results in everything we do. Fad diets feed on this desire. They make unrealistic claims that suggest that we can lose huge amounts of weight in a very short period of time "painlessly," "with no effort." If a person's goal is truly just weight loss, nothing can beat a combination of fasting and exercise. In one week's time, it might be possible to lose 10 pounds in the following way: four pounds of fat, three pounds of water, and three pounds of lean muscle tissue. But keeping this up for any length of time could be fatal. A general rule is: "The faster weight is lost, the faster it is gained back." The more radical the diet, the more anxious the dieter is to be finished with it and get back to regular eating patterns. A healthy weight loss goal is between 1 and 2 pounds a week. This enables us to take in sufficient calories to meet the body's vital requirements yet still lose weight. It is important to keep in mind that 1 to 2 pounds a week is 52 to 104 pounds a year! Anyone losing at a much faster pace than this is actually losing water, which is simply replaced later, and lean muscle tissue, which we really don't want to lose. It is not just weight we want to lose, it's fat!

Fad Diets—A Fad to Avoid

To cause weight loss, a diet must contain fewer calories than we burn. The diet can be a combination of foods, a single food, or no food at all. When nutritionists and doctors warn of the dangers inherent in many fad diets, they aren't referring to a lack of weight loss. They are referring to the danger of long-range negative effects on overall health. Fad diets that are not safe usually have one or more of these characteristics:

1. Deficient in nutrients.
2. Unbalanced in nutrients.
3. Contribute to disease and illness.
4. Cause loss of lean body tissue.

High Protein-Low Carbohydrate Diets

A diet high in protein and low in carbohydrates must be a diet high in animal products. We have already discussed the problems of this type of diet. Primarily, it contains excessive amounts of saturated fat and cholesterol, which increases the risk of heart disease. Surprisingly, this diet can also cause a loss of lean body tissue. In a balanced diet, adequate in carbohydrate and calories, protein is left to serve its main task of growth and repair. In a high-protein diet there are not enough carbohydrates available for energy, so protein must be diverted from its main function to be converted to glucose to allow the brain and nervous system to function normally. The brain always gets priority over the muscles for the available carbohydrate (glucose), since the muscles can function on fat at low levels of energy expenditure. If an individual on such a diet attempted to exercise as well (a very fatiguing feat!), the tissue loss would be even more pronounced since the requirement for glucose increases as energy demands increase.

Much of the early weight loss that occurs during a high-protein diet is actually water loss. Because the large amount of protein in the diet produces urea, large amounts of water must be taken from the body cells to dilute and eliminate the urea.

So far I have demonstrated that part of the weight loss from high-protein diets comes from two sources we don't want to lose—lean tissue and water. What about fat? On this type of diet fat is being used as the main energy source. Since fat is such a poor fuel, the dieter will feel weak, lightheaded, and fatigued. The incomplete burning of fat produces ketones, which build up in the blood and cause ketosis. Ketosis is not a healthy state, and if the blood's pH becomes too acid, serious side effects can occur. These dieters can expect to be in no physical or mental frame of mind to do much more than lie around and wonder where all their energy went.

An interesting point is that eating a diet high in protein may actually increase our craving for sweets. Drs. Judith and Richard Wurtman, cell biologists at the Massachusetts Institute of Technology, have suggested that carbohydrates release the hormone serotonin in the brain, which suppresses our desire for carbohydrates, while eating too much protein and fat actually increases our desire for carbohydrates. This may explain why people on high protein diets crave sweets and tend to go on binges, while people who eat a diet high in complex carbo-hydrates seem to be less affected by this tendency.

FASTING

Fasting has all the characteristics of the high-protein–low-carbohydrate diet, except for food. Increased lean tissue loss, dehydration, and nutrient deficiency are all symptoms of excessive fasting. During a fast, the only sources of fuel are body fat and protein, which takes us right back to ketosis again. Since fasting is even worse than the restrictive 500-calorie diets, we can assume that the stress of fasting will encourage the body to conserve fat. Once we return to a normal diet, we may find the body storing more calories than normal as fat in anticipation of another stressful fast.

LIQUID PROTEIN DIETS

The principle behind the liquid protein diet is that by taking in liquid protein we will "spare" the muscle tissue, which will not be broken down into glucose. Our major fuel source will be fat. Again, this is similar in principle to the high-protein, high-fat, low-carbohydrate diet, except that this one is even more dangerous. Several deaths have occured on this diet, although the exact cause of death was unknown. Liquid proteins are composed of incomplete proteins which lack the essential amino acids needed for tissue resynthesis. That, coupled with the fact that the diet is deficient in minerals, especially potassium and copper, may have caused the deaths.

DIET PILLS

Over-the-counter diet pills are used to suppress the appetite, which helps some people eat less. The pills have no lasting effect on weight control, only increasing our dependency on drugs to solve our problems. The multitude of testimonials from dieters which imply that the pills *caused* them to lose weight are simply misdirecting the credit. The people who lose weight and maintain that weight loss have successfully changed their eating habits. The pills did not cause the weight loss, the improvement in eating habits did.

Amphetamines and diuretics, which are obtainable only with a medical prescription, are much more dangerous than over-the-counter drugs and equally ineffective. Amphetamines are stimulants that can create a psychological dependence. The street term for amphetamines is "uppers," and that's exactly where they send the user—up the wall! Not only are they habit-forming, but they cause the user to be nervous, irritable, and at times almost irrational. Their stimulating effect on the metabolism can cause weight loss, but becoming a drug user is surely not a good long-range answer to a weight problem.

Diuretics cause water loss. Their abuse, which is common, leads to dehydration, potassium deficiency, and kidney problems. Competent doctors, who understand the principles of weight loss, will not prescribe medication for weight control unless there are extenuating medical circumstances.

STARCH BLOCKERS

The new fad of the eighties is a tablet that supposedly blocks the absorption of starches. (Starches are such foods as bread, potatoes, pastas, corn, etc.) In theory, this sounds like a great diet plan: eat all the starch you want and lose weight. In reality, it's doubtful the pills will work that way. First, they have no effect on sugars, fats, or proteins, which play a more significant role in weight control than do starches. Secondly, some users experience gas while others have experienced nausea, and there are no studies to prove or disprove their long-range health effects. At best, they appear to be dietary crutches with little support for the dieter but considerable financial support for the manufacturer. I would strongly urge you to avoid these products.

Exercises That Don't Work

SWEATING OFF FAT

Sweating off fat sounds great, but it doesn't work. Sweating causes dehydration, which is only water loss. Using methods that cause sweating simply causes water loss. Any weight loss from sweating will be replaced by drinking liquid.

Let's take an example. A person weighs 152 lbs. at 3:00 P.M., puts on a sweatsuit, and jogs for 30 minutes. That's a caloric expenditure of 14.1 calories per minute, a total of 423 calories burned. One pound of fat loss requires burning 3,500 calories. At best, only a fraction of a pound is actually lost. However, when the tired runner drags onto the scale he or she will notice a 2-pound weight loss. That loss is 2 pounds of *water*—not fat— and the weight will rapidly return. Taken to extremes, dehydration can kill. Forcing the body to heat up rapidly to cause sweating causes fatique, lack of energy, and sometimes heat prostration. To burn away fat tissue, nothing will replace exercise at a sustained pace over a long period of time. The body must give off heat. By locking in the heat with sweat suits, saunas, and excessive clothing, we reduce performance and negatively affect the body chemistry. Saunas, steam rooms, hot tubs, and whirl- pools are great for soreness or relaxing muscles—but they're useless for weight loss.

Sweat suits are often used by wrestlers, boxers, jockeys, and other athletes who are too lazy to train or diet correctly. They sometimes resort to sweating off a few pounds of water before weigh-ins, but the loss is only water; no fat reduction occurs.

Electric sweat belts are another sweat-producing gimmick. They heat up the area under the belt, stimulating perspiration in that area. Spas use these, measuring before and after use and claiming their patrons are "losing inches." The "lost inches" are only water and will almost immediately return. No loss of fat occurs.

Similar to sweat belts, waist bands are wrapped around the waist to "sweat off the fat." Forget it! It sounds logical, but our bodies don't "sweat off fat" when we are exercising. Waist bands cause a warm feeling that lets us kid ourselves that we are doing something constructive about that fat.

SPOT-REDUCING

We can't magically make fat disappear from our waists or any other area of our bodies simply by exercising that part of the body. Although any exercise burns fat, the exercising of one muscle group is insignificant compared to the exercising of the whole body. When we say the body burns fat by exercising, we don't mean that the fat on the arms feeds the arms and the fat on the waist feeds the waist. Energy expenditure draws fat from all the fat stores in the body. That is why a marathon runner doesn't just have trim legs. He or she draws from all the fat stores equally. A jogger may find the fat reducing more quickly in the arms than in the legs.

Those who have reduced overall fat can use exercise to firm and tighten specific muscles or groups of muscles. If high-resistance exercise (for example, weight training) is used, the muscles become stronger as well. Some fat loss does occur from the muscle, but the subcutaneous fat (the fat we see, found under the skin) still remains.

Spot-reducing exercises are fine for strengthening, firming, and toning muscle tissue, but only after excess fat has been lost through an aerobic exercise program.

PASSIVE EXERCISES

Passive exercises, popularly used in reducing salons, are totally useless! We must move our own bodies to burn calories. If we don't burn carlories, we won't lose fat. Anybody would be interested in the prospect of losing weight without moving, but those who just sit, stand, or lie there letting the pulleys, belts, rollers, massages, wraps, and movable tables do the work are getting ripped off. No one can rub our fat away—we have to burn it!

Another type of passive exercise is the popular muscle stimulator. Proponents suggest, for example, that just 5 minutes on the machine is equal to 200 sit-ups. Since sit-ups don't burn many calories, I doubt that such a machine can make much of a contribution to losing fat, not to mention the other hundred or so muscles in your body that need exercise! Their only usefulness may be in the rehabilitation of muscles where the individual cannot contract the muscle himself. Stay away from this kind of hoax.

HEALTH SPAS AND REDUCING SALONS

Spas don't do anything that we can't do for ourselves. The successful ones use a combination of aerobic exercise and diet control. Everything else is simply to pamper us and make us think we are getting our money's worth.

A student of mine once got very upset in class because I attacked a popular reducing salon that used movable tables. The clients lie on a table, and the machine massages different parts of their bodies. That doesn't do a thing for weight loss. The student said that I must be "nuts," because she had lost 30 pounds at this salon. What happened? She was highly motivated to lose weight. The salon gave her a 500-calorie diet and a workout program and took her $300.00. The student stuck to the diet like glue and didn't miss a workout. She lost 30 pounds which were not all fat and gave all the credit to the salon. Actually, the diet, although a poor one, caused all the weight loss; the machine did nothing.

As in most stories of this kind, the benefit from the expensive salon-reducing program was short-lived. The diet was nutritionally terrible, so the student resumed her normal eating pattern as soon as the weight was gone and promptly gained back the pounds. She has since changed her life-style to include sensible dieting and jogs three miles a day, a less expensive and more permanent solution to her weight problem.

TAKING MEASUREMENTS

Another gimmick of the reducing salon is the tape-measure trick. It is human nature to suck in the stomach and pull the tape a little tighter when measuring the waist. Ah! A trim 32″ instead of 35″! At the spa they do just the opposite. At first they say, "Relax, let it all hang out. We want a true measurement." Then they relax the tape, too. After a week of passive exercises they measure again. Wanting to be successful, the dieter doesn't stand there like a slug, but inhales and pulls in the stomach a little, never noticing that the tape's a little tighter, too. "Two inches less! You're doing great," they say. This hooks the dieter for a time, but week after week not much else happens. After all, how tight can you pull the tape? Then the guilt trip begins. "You're not doing your exercises." "Are you eating more than usual?" The dieter finally gives up and quits, a few hundred dollars poorer and feeling like a failure.

WEIGHT LIFTING

Weight lifting is not a good starting place for people who have a lot of excess weight to lose. The failure rate is extremely high. The best plan is to lose most of the fat first, then start a sensible weight-training program. As we have seen, if we increase muscle mass we increase our calorie requirements. This will have a beneficial effect, but it must be done in conjunction with an aerobic program such as walking, jogging, or cycling. I tell fat people to do such exercises first. When they have gotten most of the fat off, we start a progressive weight-training program. That's good news to them, too. They don't really want to do all that hard work anyway!

Weight Control and Athletic Performance

Athletes fall into three distinct categories with regard to weight control. The first group is interested in gaining weight. This group usually includes football players and weight sports persons (competing in discus, javelin, etc.). The second group is interested in maintaining a low weight. Wrestlers, gymnasts, and crew racers are likely to fall into this category. The third group is made up of athletes who do not feel that weight gain or loss is significant to performance.

The main concern for athletes should be the ratio of body fat to muscle mass. Two athletes can be the same weight yet have different body mass compositions. We notice instantly the visual difference between a very lean and muscular athlete of 200 pounds and a fat athlete of equal weight with flabby muscles.

Regardless of whether weight gain or loss is desired, the athlete's primary interest should be in fat, not just in total weight. A football player who gains 50 pounds isn't accomplishing much if the gain is mostly fat. On the other hand, the young gymnast who loses 20 pounds may do great harm to his or her performance and health if most of the weight loss is muscle tissue rather than fat! This is quite a common occurrence on the semi-starvation diets often employed by athletes who are trying to achieve a specific weight.

Generally speaking, a low percentage of body fat relates to better performance in all activities. Those who gain weight need to gain muscle, and those who lose need to be sure that they lose fat. Since nutrition is a major factor in energy, it is also important that the athlete approach the weight control program with his or her energy needs in mind. If the weight loss is too rapid, performance will be jeopardized by the lack of energy-producing calories. The athlete who eats too much of the wrong foods will find his or her performance impaired by a gain in fat instead of muscle. The intensive training of most athletes burns an abundance of calories. When losing weight, the athlete must avoid a reduction in calories that creates a loss of more than one-third of a pound a day. The higher the energy demand of the sport, the more caution must be taken when limiting calories.

Body Fat Versus Lean Muscle

Weight control has a direct bearing on athletic performance. If a gain in weight is the result of an increase in the amount of body fat, performance is reduced. This is especially true in endurance and high-performance events.

Generally speaking, all athletes will perform better if their percentage of body fat is low. Dr. David Costill points out that each percent increase in body fat causes an athlete's performance to decline an equal percentage point. Generally speaking, highly conditioned athletes have lower levels of body fat. Distance runners and wrestlers are often as low as 5%, football linemen about 17%, and backs about 10%. Most women athletes have a higher percentage of body fat, as do all women, than men, but there are indications that when the female body is highly trained, women may be able to reduce fat percentages to equal those of men. The optimum fat level for athletes without jeopardizing strength seems to be between 5% and 7%. Some mature, highly trained athletes have exceptionally low body fat and still perform well. Frank Shorter, a world class marathoner, has only 3% body fat. Some Olympic wrestlers have between 2% and 3%, and a few very muscular football players are equally low.

Power Sports: Adding Muscle or Fat?

Power sports are activities such as football, hockey, weight events (discus and shot), and heavy-weight wrestling, where there are no limitations on size. The more mass put on the line or behind the throw, the better the performance. Since power athletes can't do anything about their height, they quite logically concentrate on their weight. The more, the better! Resistive weight training, accompanied by more calories, will put on weight. The question is, "Do we really want more weight or do we want more muscle?" Obviously, the athlete wants more muscle, which will result in more mass and strength. Unhappily, what many get is not enough muscle (from weight training) and too much fat (from too many calories).

Take, for example, two football linemen who start identically with body fat at 15% and weight at 210 pounds. They both gain 40 pounds during the year from an intensive weight program. By visual observations, we may not notice much difference between the two, but if we can measure their percentage of body fat we can get a more exact picture of their weight gain. After training, player "A" is found to have 15% body fat, while player "B" has 20%. Player "A" has gained 32 pounds of muscle mass and only 6 pounds of fat. Player "B" has gained the same amount of weight with only 20 pounds being muscle and 20 pounds being fat.

EXAMPLE:

Start:

Both players: 210 pounds, 15% fat (31 pounds fat, 181 pounds lean mass)

After Weight Training:

Player "A": 250 pounds, 15% fat (37 pounds fat, 213 pounds lean mass)

Player "B": 250 pounds, 20% fat (50 pounds fat, 200 pounds lean mass)

Player "A" has a much greater probability of performing well on the field than player "B." Since in this case they both followed the same weight program, it was the diet that caused player "B" to gain so much fat. Excessive calories, accompanied by more protein than his muscles could utilize, put on fat. Player "A" ate only the calories and protein required for energy expenditure and tissue development.

Gaining weight does have its limitations. Power athletes who gain excessive weight, regardless of whether it's muscle or fat, can be endangering their health. It is not uncommon to see very large athletes suffer from hypertension, high cholesterol, and other cardiac risk factors.

In time, the use of body fat measurements will replace the scale. Power athletes will realize that low body fat correlates to a high performance level and better health. Suppose for a moment that one of our football players increased his weight from 210 pounds to 230 pounds instead of 250 pounds, decreasing his body fat to only 10%. This would have resulted in only 6 pounds less lean mass, but 14 pounds less extra fat. Carrying 14 pounds less fat would cause an improvement in overall performance.

Power athletes will better their results if they will reduce body fat through a positive diet and aerobic training, while maintaining an adequate resistive weight-training program.

Weight Reduction Sports

The need for weight loss is most common in sports such as wrestling, rowing, boxing, and gymnastics. Anyone considering a weight-reduction program should first know his or her percentage of body fat. A wrestler weighing 130 pounds would be hard pressed to make the 118-pound class if he had only 5% body fat. That's only 6½ pounds of fat. If he lost 3 pounds of fat, he would be down to a bare minimum of only 3% body fat at 127 pounds. Any additional loss would have to come from lean body tissue and/or dehydration, both of which would impair his performance and endanger his health. The problem we are faced with today is the wrestler who is either too lazy or not knowledgeable enough about nutrition to lose weight correctly.

It is not uncommon to see a wrestler drop from 130 pounds to 118 pounds in less than a week. Even with the most rigorous training schedule, this wrestler could not lose more than 2 to 4 pounds of actual fat. The additional 8 to 10 pounds is mostly water and some muscle tissue. This loss is accomplished by starvation, exercise, and, during the last day or so, by total dehydration using saunas, sweat suits, and, finally, spitting! By weigh-in time, this wrestler can expect his carbohydrate reserves to be depleted, and he will experience dehydration, fatigue, lassitude, and a noncompetitive attitude. After weigh-in, he will load up on food, water, supplements, or anything else he thinks might help him to regain his competitive level of fitness. As we have already learned, by this time it's too late! The body simply cannot be rehydrated and the energy storages rebuilt in a few hours. That takes days. The best this wrestler can hope for is that his opponent cut his weight the same way (highly probable) or that he's more skilled than his opponent.

A much better approach, but one that requires self-discipline, is practicing positive nutrition with an emphasis on losing weight over a longer period of time. At 130 pounds and 15% body fat, we can expect any athlete to reduce to an excellent 117 pounds with 5% body fat in only seven weeks.

To lose two pounds a week (recommended) would require a reduction of 7,000 calories (3,500 = 1 pound). This can be accomplished by a daily 1,000-calorie reduction. For hard-training athletes who consume in excess of 3,000 calories a day, this reduction would still leave over 2,000 calories, which is sufficient for endurance training. Following a 7-week program, an athlete should be able to drop to 117 pounds. We can assume that while he or she loses 13 pounds of fat, the athlete will probably gain a few pounds of muscle tissue as a result of the training program. That would put his or her weight at 120 pounds with 5% body fat. If the athlete can maintain that weight throughout the season, he or she will have no problem losing the two to three pounds prior to competition. He or she will give a peak performance and, more importantly, will be training at an optimum level.

Testing for Body Fat

All coaches should have their teams tested to determine body fat ratio on a regular basis. Any local college that has a tank can be contacted to see if they will test the team. If they cannot do it for free, they will probably do it for a nominal fee. If that is inconvenient, the skin calipers are very adequate.

Measurement before and after a weight-loss or -gain program is very important. If a football player is measured at 10% body fat before he starts lifting weights, we can measure him periodically to be sure that his gain is muscle, not fat. If it stays steady, we know the gain is muscle.

Ideally, athletes should talk about their percentage of body fat and lean muscle mass rather than about their weight. Someday, perhaps, sportscasters will announce at football games the lean body weight of the front line rather than the weight. It sounds unequal when they announce "South High with a front line weighing 250 pounds against North High with a line weighing 230 pounds." But if South High's line has 20% body fat and North High's has only 10%, the call should sound like this: "South High with a front line weighing 200 lbs. of lean muscle mass agains North High with a front line weighing 207 pounds of lean muscle mass." All things being equal, North High would be the best bet. That 50 pounds of fat will take its toll in the fourth quarter.

Questions and Answers

Q: *Is there a danger in being overweight?*
A: The danger of excess weight lies in its relationship to other diseases. For that reason it is a disease in itself. Being excessively overweight (20% or more) predisposes you to heart disease, stroke, diabetes, gallstones, degenerative joint disease, high cholesterol, high blood pressure, and, for women the added risk of uterine cancer. To all of this we can add the reduction in energy level that prevents many overweight people from true enjoyment of their work and play. Government statistics indicate that if everyone were of optimal weight, there would be 25% less heart disease and 35% fewer strokes (blockage of brain vessels).

Q: *Isn't overweight caused by heredity and other factors?*
A: Some is. Maybe 5% can be attributed to heredity, hormone imbalance, or other disorders. Whether these conditions trigger overweight or the overweight triggers them is still not certain. But about 95% of all overweight is caused by too little exercise and/or overeating.

Q: *Don't some people have more "fat cells," which makes it impossible to lose weight?*
A: Infants and adolescents who are overfed may develop more fat cells than normal. This can result in a greater tendency to be overweight later in life. It may be more difficult to lose weight, but it's not impossible.

Q: *I've heard that they have discovered an enzyme deficiency in obese people.*
A: Doctors at Beth Israel Hospital in Boston found a deficiency of an enzyme called sodium-potassium ATPase in obese patients. This enzyme acts as the "sodium pump," letting potassium into the cells and keeping sodium out. It is believed that 30% to 40% of the energy in the body is spent maintaining this balance. Although this is still theory, I'm sure that *some* obese people have internal malfunctions that they are unaware of. Most, however, simply eat too much.

Q: *How low can I go on my calorie intake while dieting to lose weight?*

158

A: I suggest you go no lower than 1,200 calories. This will have the least effect on your metabolism and health. Drop your food intake 300 to 500 calories and exercise enough to burn 300 to 500 calories.

Q: *Can I get fat without gaining weight?*
A: You can actually get fat without gaining weight! This happens because fat is stored inside the muscles, not just under the skin. When the muscles start to atrophy due to inactivity, fat is exchanged for the muscle tissue. This commonly occurs as people get older. They often "get fat" even though there is no significant weight change. Their body-fat weight goes up as their lean-body weight goes down, changing their ratio of body fat, but not their total weight.

Q: *Do women have more problems with weight loss?*
A: Yes. Women always have a higher percent of body fat which means less lean tissue to feed, so their calorie requirements are less. Most women in my classes want to lose weight when actually all they need is exercise, which will cause some fat loss, but more importantly will exchange fat for muscle. Often, women who want to go from 120 pounds to 110 pounds actually only need to eliminate fat and replace it with muscle. At 110 pounds they may look sickly and underweight.

Q: *Do you need more calories if you're fat?*
A: No. You need fewer calories if you're fat, since lean body mass, not the fat, uses most of the calories. If you're 200 pounds and 30% fat, your lean mass is 140 pounds and your fat is 60 pounds. Your 140 pounds, not your 60 pounds of fat, uses most of your calories. On the other hand, if you're only 10% fat, like some football players, you're feeding 180 pounds of lean mass and carrying 20 pounds of fat. You may weigh 200 pounds, but you don't feed 200 pounds. Feed that smaller person inside (lean body mass).

Q: *Then if you had more lean mass you could eat more?*
A; Yes. By being overweight and sedentary, you lose muscle mass. Fat people are really feeding smaller people inside! If you increase your lean muscle mass and lose fat you can normalize your calorie requirements much more easily. Calorie require-

ments usually go up after you bring your body fat percentage down.

Q: *Should I take vitamins and minerals when I diet?*
A: Yes. A good multi-vitamin-mineral supplement is advisable when total calorie intake is reduced.

Q: *Do we have the same calorie needs, based on weight, throughout life?*
A: No. It is generally estimated that one's calorie needs are reduced 5% every decade after the age of 20. This is true for most people because of a loss in lean body mass as a result of a more sedentary life-style. If people were more active, this drop would not occur. Jack LaLanne, the T.V. exercise host, is about 70 years of age and still has the physique of a 20-year-old athlete.

Q: *I want to lose weight faster than one pound a week.*
A: The one-pound recommendation is best because it avoids radical diet adjustments. The heavier you are, the more you will lose per week. An aerobic exercise program coupled with a caloric restriction is the ideal way to lose weight. To lose much over 2 to 3 pounds a week would mean a loss of water and lean muscle tissue. If you feel you must lose more, do it only under strict medical supervision.

Q: *Are there specific foods that are fattening?*
A: Not really. It's density that you're concerned with. You can put 1,000 calories of ice cream in one good-sized bowl, but 1,000 calories of mixed vegetables would fill several large bowls. Don't exceed your total calorie need, and make sure you're meeting your nutritional requirements. One hundred calories of ice cream is the same as one hundred calories of vegetables.

Q: *Could I lose weight on a diet of junk food?*
A: Yes, if you were on a restricted calorie intake. You could also lose your life. Malnutrition would be the result of an extended time on a junk-food diet. The weight you lost would just be gained back, anyway, when you returned to your normal eating pattern.

Q: *What about the new fat clubs? They say fat is beautiful.*
A: Only you can decide what is beautiful to you. You may be able to stay somewhat "plump" and feel fine. Our concern with excessive overweight is disease, not vanity. People who belong to "fat clubs" are usually very obese. I think they have given up on themselves. Once you consciously give up on anything, you try to justify it by reducing its importance. I have *never* met an obese person who was not healthier and happier after they lost the excess weight. Self-image is a major motivator, but good health is the bottom line.

Q: *When you suggest walking for exercise, does that include walking while shopping?*
A: No. Strolling with your boyfriend or girlfriend also doesn't count. The heart rate doesn't go up enough (at least not from the walk!). I mean walking at a good pace. After a while you will be able to walk very briskly. You may then want to start jogging to speed the burning of calories.

Q: *I don't have time to walk.*
A: Do you have time to die? Make time! You wouldn't be reading this book if you didn't want to lose weight and be healthy. Movement is very natural to the human body.

Q: *What is cellulite?*
A: Those who believe in cellulite want you to believe that it's a special type of fat that responds only to special methods of removal. Cellulite is the term used for flabby portions of the body that have an "orange peel" appearance. It is common among women, and it has more to do with skin type than the fat under the skin.

Spas charge exorbitant prices for women to be wrapped in plastic and massaged, which is supposed to eliminate cellulite. At best this draws water out of the tissue, which is simply replaced later. People who follow a healthy diet and exercise aerobically will control fat, cellulite, or whatever else people choose to call it.

Q: *If I weigh myself, will that tell me the amount of fat I'm losing?*

A: No—only the total amount of weight you have lost. We all like to look at the scale just to see what's happening, but a true picture will be found only in a test of body fat.

Q: *Where do I get a body-fat test?*
A: A doctor interested in physical fitness can direct you to a laboratory available to the community. At our college we have a physical performance laboratory where you can get a body-fat test. Using the hydrostatic (underwater immersion) weight measurement, we can get the most accurate test for body fat. The skin-fold test is a second good choice.

Q: *Is grapefruit a fat eliminator?*
A: No. The grapefruit diet claimed that enzymes in grapefruit "mobilize" fat. There is no evidence for this in nutritional literature. Grapefruit is fine to eat, but don't expect it to cause a reduction in fat tissue.

Q: *How can I "spare" the protein I eat so that it will be used for tissue replacement?*
A: Eat enough other calories to meet your energy demands. The best calories for energy are natural carbohydrates. A good balance of these not only reduces the breakdown of protein into glucose, it also reduces your overall protein requirements.

Q: *How do I gain weight?*
A: I assume that you want to gain lean muscle tissue, not just weight! Resistive exercise such as weight training will best stimulate muscle growth. All exercise involving total body movement stimulates muscle tissue, but to a lesser degree. Exercise is the first and most important step.

The only dietary adjustment needed to gain weight would be an increase in calories to meet the exercise demands. Eat more of the higher-calorie complex carbohydrates like whole grains, legumes, and starchy vegetables (corn, sweet potato). Do not make these mistakes:

1. Don't eat a high-protein diet or use protein supplements.
2. Don't eat high-calorie sugar foods (pies, malts, cakes).

Once your body uses the protein it needs and burns the sugar for fuel, the excess will become fat weight!

Q: *If I jog, am I burning away fat?*
A: Yes, but carbohydrates are being burned, too. If you're breathing hard during exercise you are using more carbohydrates (from the "glucose tank"). If you slow your pace so that your breathing is reduced, your fat utilization increases. Go for longer periods and fat utilization increases still further. Remember, go longer and slower for optimum fat burning.

Q: *I'm fat. I go out and run around the track two times as fast as I can, rest, and then do it again. What do you think?*
A: Since you are going full speed, your oxygen uptake is maximal. You're burning almost 100% glucose. That fat guy jogging slowly around the track is burning more fat than you are. Join him and get the fat off! Leave the speed for when your body is lean and well trained.

Q: *Are you saying it's a waste of time to run fast since you burn only carbohydrates?*
A: Only at first. As you lose weight (fat) and get into condition you utilize oxygen better, thus burning more fat. A marathon runner utilizes oxygen very well, which allows him to burn fat and spare glucose.

Q: *I think I'm one of those people who's getting fatter but not gaining weight. I look and feel heavier.*
A: Your muscles and other tissues have sucked up a great deal of fat. They are similar to marbled meat (found in sedentary cattle or people). You have lost muscle tissue (atrophy due to no physical stress) and replaced it with fat. Since fat is lighter than muscle, you can take on more fat. You look heavier but you're not. You're just fatter!

Q: *Would we be right in saying that most overweight people need to increase their lean body mass as well as reduce their fat mass?*
A: Right on! Diet and exercise both play a role, but *only exercise* can increase lean mass. Without the stimulus of exercise, calories go to fat.

Q: *I saw a beautiful movie star on T.V. who gave all the credit for her weight loss to a "cellulite" removal program at a Beverly Hills salon.*

A: Being beautiful and a movie star does not bestow nutritional and physiological expertise. Her own motivation toward a sound diet and exercise caused her to lose the cellulite, not the $1,000 she paid the salon!

Q: *You mentioned that people who exercise aerobically burn more fat. Where do these runners get their fat? They're so skinny!*
A: Remember that fat is highly concentrated. One pound has 3,500 calories. An athlete who weighs 140 pounds and only has 3% body fat has 4 pounds of fat or 14,000 calories of stored fat. A runner who runs under five minutes per mile will burn about 1,200 calories an hour. Since part of the fuel comes from glucose, it's impossible for him or her to use up the 14,000 calories of fat. This fat is hidden inside the active muscles; it doesn't hang around the body like it does in nonathletes.

Q: *I hate to exercise. How do I lose weight?*
A: By diet alone, but it's very slow and difficult. Once you lose the weight you will find it difficult to prevent a weight gain unless you do some type of exercise to stimulate your metabolism.

Q: *What's wrong with the radical diet, if you can lose weight fast?*
A: The same thing that's wrong with using drugs to feel good all the time—the side effects! Think of how you can lose weight permanently. Losing weight without making lifelong dietary changes is just a waste of effort. The weight will come right back.

Q: *Why is slow weight loss the best way?*
A: It means you have made a psychological commitment to weight loss and are willing to change your bad habits. Anyone can go on a crash diet for one or two weeks, as long as they know they can go back to their regular habits. The same is true of smoking, drinking, etc.

Q: *Are there people who should not go on a diet?*
A: Yes. Anyone who is not psychologically committed to the personal value of weight loss.

Q: *If I have a low percentage of body fat and still think I'm fat, what should I do?*
A: Exercise to gain muscle mass. All exercise will increase muscle mass, but resistive weight training does it the best.

Q: *What is anorexia?*
A: An obsessive desire to avoid eating at any cost to the health. Its roots are probably more psychological than physiological. It's common among teen-age girls who have an obsession with extreme weight loss. Being skinny is the ultimate goal. They should be directed to professional psychological help.

Q: *Can I eat sweets and still lose weight?*
A: Yes. Small amounts of sweets can be accommodated in an otherwise well-balanced, low-calorie diet. If you're eating 1,200 calories a day to lose weight, 100 calories of sweets can be part of that total.

Q: *What food should I avoid?*
A: Nothing. Identify the foods *you* eat that contribute the most calories to your diet and eat less of them. Obviously, eliminating the fattening foods might be best; but if you feel that it is too much of a sacrifice, eat small amounts of them.

Q: *What complex carbohydrates should I curtail in a weight-loss program?*
A: Watch your intake of grains, legumes, nuts, avocados, and high-starch foods like corn and sweet potatoes. Don't eliminate them, just don't go overboard.

Q: *How can whole-grain bread be less fattening than white bread?*
A: It isn't, but because it has more fiber it's more filling. An open-faced sandwich using one slice of whole-grain bread is more filling than a sandwich made with two slices of white bread, with a net savings of 175 calories.

Q: *What's a simple way to cut calories when shopping, without converting grams to calories?*
A: Avoid canned and highly processed food. Shop in the produce section and buy fresh meat, fish, and poultry. That's an oversimplification, but I think you get the point.

Q: *What about behavior modification for weight control?*
A: If you refer to the idea of associating when, where, and how to eat, and then changing these situations, I can't say that I'm too excited about the long-range prospects. Most people simply are

not aware of their bad habits and do not understand nutrition sufficiently to make correct choices. Other people just don't care.

Q: *Don't some people have a real obsession with food, which makes it difficult for them to discipline their dietary habits?*
A: Yes. Their association with food is much stronger than just a need for nutrients and energy. They place too much emphasis on food as a reward mechanism to make them happy. They easily justify eating binges as being associated with happiness and the fun of life. These individuals should seek psychological counseling to cure their obsession with food. Knowing the right way to eat is only half the battle for them.

Q: *Isn't eating a social function for all of us?*
A: Yes. But the purpose isn't to eat yourself into oblivion. It's to have social interaction with other people. Food can enhance the social situation without becoming the prime objective.

Q: *It's hard to avoid overeating in social situations. I seem to just keep eating and eating at parties. What can I do?*
A: Try to look at it the same way you look at social drinking. Most people learn to control their drinking in social situations to avoid getting drunk and having a hangover. They learn to recognize their limits and control their intake. If you will apply that same principle to eating, you will learn a good lesson in self-discipline.

Q: *It's really a drag to discipline yourself all the time. It's more fun to eat and drink.*
A: The basic rule in our environment is "There's no such thing as a free lunch." Applied to overeating, that means that if you eat to excess without regard for your health or weight, you will undoubtedly suffer for it later in life. Look at the long-range effect of your dietary habits rather than the immediate enjoyment of the food.

Q: *Shouldn't we enjoy eating?*
A: Yes. But every meal doesn't have to be a social occasion. There are many times when you should eat lightly just to fulfill your nutritional needs and hunger. By doing this you may find that those special meals when you eat a little more and have some

social interaction are more enjoyable and become something to look forward to.

Q: *I have trouble avoiding ice cream. I love it! What should I do?*
A: Include it in your diet on a limited basis rather than as a regular daily habit. You'll find you can function quite well without it and will enjoy it more on the occasions you do eat it.

Q: *I'm lifting weights and increasing my calorie intake to gain 20 pounds. How do I know if I'm gaining muscle or fat?*
A: Have your body fat percentage calculated before starting your program. As you gain weight, have it checked again periodically to ensure that the percentage of body fat does not go up.

Q: *I wrestle in the 190-pound class, but I notice that my weight is dropping. Should I drop down to the next weight class?*
A: First, know your body fat ratio. Drop down only if you can safely do so without your body fat going below about 5%.

Q: *Don't football players need extra fat for protection?*
A: I'm not really sure. Just because linemen statistically have a higher percentage of body fat than backs doesn't mean it's the best situation. Some great backs have as little as 3% body fat, and they get hit harder than anyone!

Q: *Do you think a 250-pound tackle with 20% fat should lose weight?*
A: Yes. At 250 pounds he's carrying 50 pounds of fat. If he lost 20 pounds of fat, he would reduce his percent of fat to about 13% and still maintain 200 pounds of lean body mass and a total weight of 230 pounds. I think he will have more endurance and speed and show an improvement in total performance.

Q: *Doesn't an increase in body mass have some positive value to football players?*
A: Yes. But keep as much mass as possible in the form of muscle rather than fat. Let's put it another way. As a coach I'd rather have a football player who weighs 250 pounds with a body fat ratio of 13% than one that has 20% fat. Less fat means more efficiency.

Q: *If exercise increases muscle mass won't my muscles get too big?*
A: No. It takes high-resistance weight training to develop a high degree of muscle mass. The muscle stimulation you get from walking and jogging will not be accentuated by large bulging muscles. You have to really work intensively in a weight-lifting program to get the larger, stronger muscles common in strength athletes.

Q: *Which is more important in weight control, diet or exercise?*
A: Probably exercise, but a combination is best because most people do not want to spend a great amount of time exercising.

Q: *How effective is dieting without exercise?*
A: Only about 10% of obese people are able to lose weight and keep it off without exercising. I personally doubt that they will look that great even at a reduced weight due to the flabbiness of their muscle tissue.

Q: *Can the type of food you eat affect your weight even if the calories are the same?*
A: Maybe. Dr. Otho E. Michaelis IV, of the U.S. Department of Agriculture, fed animals equal diets except that one group got 54% of its carbohydrates from starch and the other 54% from sucrose. The group on sucrose had a 35% weight gain and more fat tissue. They also showed signs of adult diabetes and high serum triglycerides. If the same thing applies to humans, then it supports the recommendation that we eat less sucrose.

Q: *Can reducing my body fat and increasing my muscle mass really improve my athletic performance?*
A: Definitely. I've seen many athletes improve their performance just through nutrition, jogging, and weight training. The sad story is that of the athletes who find out too late. I wish I had a nickel for every athlete who said "I wish I knew this when I was in high school."

Q: *I'm a wrestler. Should I gain weight through weight training and go up a weight class or lose fat and go down a weight class?*
A: Wrestle at the weight you can perform at optimally. First, keep your body fat low, at perhaps 5% to 8%. If you're not strong

enough, lift weights. If that moves you up a weight class without increasing your fat percentage, then you may perform better. Always improve your weakest link. When I was coaching I had a 126-pounder who took sixth in the state because he wasn't very strong. By going on a strength program he gained muscle mass, went up to 150 pounds in his sophomore year, and placed second in the state. Wrestling a lower weight class is only productive if you don't sacrifice strength and endurance.

8
MAKING POSITIVE NUTRITIONAL SELECTIONS

Which Diet is Best?

It seems that everyone is looking for a diet to serve a specific purpose. The overweight frantically jump from one diet to another in the hope of finding the best weight-loss diet, while the youth-seekers are eager to add or delete any food or food group they think will keep them young. Let's face it, there are no absolutes! We can't say that this diet or that diet is the best for everyone. However, we do know that the closer we can come to a natural diet, the healthier we will be. Scientists may not have all the answers yet, but they're on the right track. The "best" weight-loss diet is a healthy diet that becomes part of the life-style. The same is true of "stay younger diets," "heart diets," and all the others aimed at a longer, healthier life.

As I have pointed out in this book, obesity, overweight, heart disease, and probably countless other illnesses (including the loss of youth) can be attributed, at least in part, to dietary abuses. Poor diet increases the chances of falling prey to any number of illnesses.

Positive nutrition contributes to our total well-being. For some this may mean a vegetarian diet. For many it may include animal products. Remember, no absolutes! What we are attempting to do in this chapter is to give guidelines for positive nutrition that will help control weight and contribute to prevention of disease.

Each person must decide how many of the recommendations to adopt. For example, no one can guarantee that reducing your fat intake to 10% of your total calories will protect you from heart disease, but there is no question that you should eat less fat. Each individual must evaluate his or her own diet and then decide if there is value in making a change.

Keeping in mind that there are no absolutes, it is not necessary to change all of our eating habits overnight. Any change for the better is progress. We mustn't add stress to life by feeling guilty over eating a food that is unhealthful. However, we do need to develop a conscience to urge us to continue to eliminate the foods that we know are bad for us. It is important to care about good health!

There are no hard and fast rules for improving nutrition. We simply must keep trying to improve each week, each month, and each year. It's where we're going that counts, not how long it takes to get there. The prize is improved health!

COMPARING TWO DIETS

Many of us make very poor decisions in our daily food selections without giving much thought to their total effect on our health. Below is a daily food intake that would lead to poor health if it became a typical dietary habit. I'm sure most of you will recognize it!

BREAKFAST
3-egg omelette and cheese
4 strips of bacon
Hash browns with butter

BREAKFAST (continued)

1 glass of whole milk
2 slices of white bread

LUNCH (Fast Food Restaurant)

Double cheeseburger
Vanilla shake
French fries

DINNER (Fast Food Restaurant)

Fried Chicken Dinner:
3 pieces of chicken
Mashed potatoes and gravy
Cole slaw
White roll

Everyone's diet varies, but this is fairly typical. Some people start with eggs instead of an omelette or eat a top sirloin steak instead of the hamburger, but that doesn't change things very much. Others, of course, substitute a Danish pastry, hot dogs, sloppy Joes, pizza, and an array of other "foods," all of which have the same negative effect.

Let's evaluate the effects of this diet on one's health:

Fat: This diet is not only too high in fat but is especially high in saturated fat, which helps to clog our arteries and reduce the efficient flow of oxygen to the cells.

Carbohydrate: No one would win a marathon on this low-carbohydrate diet! The energy source is too dependent on fat and protein, which cause sluggishness. The main carbohydrates are refined sugar and white flour. About one-third of the carbohydrate intake is from refined sugar. Even those who wanted to exercise to lose weight would find it difficult on these poor fuel sources.

Protein: This diet contains well over 100 grams of protein. This will cause the kidneys to work overtime trying to eliminate the excess urea. What the system can't eliminate will be converted to fat. Most of the protein is animal protein, which increases saturated-fat intake, and since the total protein intake is so high it's possible that calcium absorption is low and phosphorus intake is high. This causes an imbalance of the two minerals.

Cholesterol: If the cholesterol theory is right these people are in big trouble. This diet is extremely high in cholesterol (close to 1,000 milligrams) because of the high animal-food content. The chicken dinner was a good idea, but when it is deep-fried (probably in palm oil), it absorbs too much fat and too many calories to remain a healthy choice. With this diet there's a good chance that the arteries will become occluded in later life—if there is a later life.

Fiber: This diet is very low in fiber. There is no fiber in the animal products, and the very small amount of carbohydrates (toast, potatoes, roll, and cole slaw) are all highly processed, which means much of the fiber is removed in milling.

Vitamins and Minerals: Some of the important vitamins and minerals are present, but it is doubtful if the balance of trace minerals, other essential B vitamins, and vitamin C are adequate.

Salt: This diet is so high in salt that a blood pressure test once a week would be a good idea. A diagnosis of hypertension should be anticipated as a result of this diet.

All of this paints a pretty bleak picture. Obviously, not all of us eat like this, but those who do can expect disease and poor health. We all need to evaluate our own diets, determine how much of this scenario applies to us, and begin to develop a better eating pattern.

A better selection might look something like this:

BREAKFAST

Bowl of grapenuts with skim milk
Sliced banana
1 glass of fresh orange juice
2 slices whole-grain toast and jam

SNACK

Whole fruit (apple, pear, etc.)
Nonfat yogurt

LUNCH

½-Tuna sandwich on whole-grain bread
Tossed green salad (mixed)
Small lentil soup
Cantaloupe slices
1 glass of nonfat milk

SNACK

Whole fruit
Whole-grain crackers

DINNER

Spaghetti with clams (whole-grain pasta—low-oil sauce)
Whole-grain rolls with butter
Tossed green salad
Small amount of steamed vegetables
White wine

SNACK

Sliced fresh fruit

This diet is much healthier. You can control the calories simply by adjusting the size of the portions. The first thing we notice is that it's low in animal products, which reduces cholesterol, total fat, and saturated fat. The tuna, clams, nonfat milk, and yogurt make up the total animal food. This is far less than the eggs, bacon, cheese, meat, whole milk, and fried chicken found in the first example. The carbohydrates are much more nutritious, since they are derived from natural complex carbohydrates. Fruit, whole-grain cereal, pasta, and bread, along with lentils and other mixed vegetables, make up most of the carbohydrates, which are also high in fiber. The protein content is relatively low due to the lower intake of animal foods. Since salt is not added to any of the food, the salt content is naturally occurring in most of the foods; but this can vary depending on whether food is homemade or eaten at a restaurant.

Don't assume that the first example is a totally poor selection or that the second one is ideal. You could mix some of the items from each and come up with a pretty good alternative menu. A poached egg now and then in place of cereal is fine; a hamburger (small) on a whole-grain bun with salad and fruit is enjoyable and nutritious. The fried chicken can become skinned breast of chicken with mushrooms and a low-fat sauce. Many changes can be made in your food selection that will improve your health and still be enjoyable. Nutrition depends not so much on what you eat once in a while as on what you eat on a regular basis.

Characteristics of Positive Nutrition

Generally speaking, there are two things that will improve anyone's diet: eating fewer animal products high in saturated fat and eating more naturally occurring complex carbohydrates.

CHARACTERISTICS OF POSITIVE NUTRITION

A. *Percent of calories from each group:*
   Protein   10%–12%
   Carbohydrates   60%–80%
   Fat   10%–20%
B. *Specific Characteristics:*
   1. *Low in Cholesterol*
      Eat fewer animal products. Consume less than 300 mgs. of cholesterol a day.
   2. *Low in Fat*
      Eating fewer animal products will lower the saturated fat content of the diet. Less oils, butter, margarine, and lard will reduce the total fat.
   3. *Low in Protein, Especially Animal Protein*
      Eat less animal protein. Substitute plant foods (grains and legumes) for part of the protein requirement.
   4. *Low in Refined Sugar*
      No more than 10% of the total calorie intake should be refined sugar products.

5. *High in Natural Complex Carbohydrates*
   Eat more plant foods (vegetables, fruits, and grains).
6. *Low in Food Additives*
   Reduce processed foods that are high in additives.
7. *High in Fiber*
   A diet high in natural carbohydrates and low in animal products assures adequate fiber intake.
8. *Low in Salt*
   Don't add salt to food. Avoid processed foods with added salt.
9. *Low in Calories*
   Eating a high-carbohydrate, low-fat, low-protein diet makes it easier to control calorie intake. Eat enough calories to meet daily energy demands.

The Food Groups

Each group of foods has certain advantages and disadvantages. Evaluating these characteristics will help determine how much of each group to include in the diet.

MEAT, FISH, POULTRY, AND DAIRY PRODUCTS

Advantages	Disadvantages
Excellent source of protein	Contain cholesterol
Good source of vitamins and minerals	Higher in saturated fats than plant food
	No fiber
	No carbohydrates
	High in calories if fatty cuts or high-fat dairy products

The main advantage of these foods is that they are all complete proteins. From there on, it's all downhill! We need very small amounts of them to get our daily protein requirement. For example:

3 oz. meat-fish-poultry = 21 grams
1 oz. cheese = 7 grams

1 cup milk	=	9 grams
1 cup cottage cheese	=	34 grams
1 egg	=	6 grams

Imagine that, at one meal, eating a 10 ounce top sirloin steak contributes about 70 grams of protein. That comes close to meeting total protein requirements for two days! Unfortunately, the body can't store protein to be used the following day. We should eat small amounts each day. Our intake of most animal foods should be reduced. Emphasis should be on fish and poultry breasts, which are higher in polyunsaturated fats and lower in calories than the red meats. A small amount of animal protein in a diet that contains plenty of plant proteins (beans, peas, and whole grains) is totally adequate for good health.

DRIED BEANS AND PEAS

Advantages	Disadvantages
Good protein source	Poorly assimilated protein source when eaten separately
No cholesterol	
Low fat (high in polyunsaturates)	Bioavailability of minerals may be low .
High in complex carbohydrate	(Legumes and grains should be eaten together for the highest amino acid assimilation)
High in fiber	
High in vitamins and minerals	

Often regarded as the poor person's protein, beans and peas are high-quality protein that can replace much, if not all, of our animal protein. One-half cup of most legume varieties yields about 7 grams of protein, which we can exchange for about 1 ounce of animal protein.

The quality of legumes as a protein source is enhanced when we eat them with grain products (combining rice and beans, tortillas and beans, etc.). This group is very economical, low in calories compared to animal protein, and highly nutritious. As we reduce our intake of animal products, we should substitute more beans and peas to meet daily protein requirements.

GRAINS

Advantages	Disadvantages
Moderate source of protein	For best protein assimilation, eat with other protein foods
High in complex carbohydrates	Poor absorption of minerals
Small amounts fat (highly poly-unsaturated)	
No cholesterol	
High in fiber	
High in vitamins and minerals (especially vitamin B)	

Grains are the main staple of most of the world. We should select a variety of whole grains in the form of breads, cereals, pastas, rice, and whole-wheat flour products. Those who are concerned with calories can reduce the number of servings.

FRUITS AND VEGETABLES

Advantages	Disadvantages
No cholesterol	Low protein source when eaten separately
High in complex carbohydrates	Some are high in sugars
Very low in fat	
High in fiber	
High in vitamins and minerals	

Emphasize fruits and vegetables in your daily diet. Concentrate on eating more whole fruits and raw vegetables in mixed salad. Steam vegetables to enhance the quality of your diet without adding excessive calories.

NUTS AND SEEDS

Advantages	Disadvantages
Good source of vitamins and minerals	High in fat
No cholesterol	High in calories
Moderate fiber	

Nuts are mostly fat, a significant drawback.

EGGS

Advantages	Disadvantages
Excellent source of protein	Very high in cholesterol
High in vitamins and minerals	High in fat
	No fiber
	No carbohydrates

One egg yolk contains 250 milligrams of cholesterol. Egg whites are cholesterol-free. Many other foods can supply vitamins, minerals, and protein.

The Problems of Selecting from the Four Basic Food Groups

Americans are sadly lacking in nutritional information. Those who do pay attention to nutrition usually believe that they should select from the four basic food groups.

Meat and meat substitutes	2 servings
Milk and milk products	2 servings
Fruits and vegetables	4 servings
Grains (bread and cereal products)	4 servings

Unfortunately, assuming that people will make sound selections from the four basic groups borders on naiveté. Here is the way a young football player, for example, would be likely to choose:

Meat Group	2 servings: "quarter-pounder" with cheese; 3 eggs
Milk Group	2 servings: chocolate milkshake; 1 glass whole milk; 1 dish ice cream
Fruits and Vegetables	4 servings: cherry pie; apple turnover; serving of canned peas; serving of canned carrots
Grains (bread, cereal)	4 servings: bread in quarter-pounder, pie

The point is that most foods don't fit into a single category. Pizza, pies, baked goods, canned dinners, etc. are all mixtures of foods from more than one group. If we select natural foods, the basic-four plan isn't too bad as a selection guide; but without a good understanding of foods, many consumers make very poor selections.

Guidelines for Food Selection

It is difficult, if not impossible, to give a simple guideline for food selection that is adequate for everyone. We all have different likes and dislikes; therefore, it's important to have guidelines rather than inflexible rules. The following guidelines indicate the natural foods we should include in our diet:

SELECTING A DAILY DIET

1. *Meat:* Lean cuts (includes chicken and turkey breast); fish; and mixed legumes and whole grains 2–3 times a week. — 1–2 servings

2. *Dairy products:* Low-fat products only. Dairy products can substitute for some of the meat group. — 1–2 servings

3. *Whole fruit:* One citrus fruit and three others. Choose fresh fruits. — 2–4 servings daily

   Vegetables: Mixture of raw and steamed. Include dark green and yellow varieties. — 2–4 servings daily

4. *Whole grains:* Variety of grains (rice, cereals, breads, pasta, flours). — 2–4 servings daily

5. *Avoid fats and oils:* Essential oils are found in natural grains and other plant foods. — Minimal amount should be served as salad dressings, spreads, whole-grain products

The following chart will provide a quick reference for food selection. The less we eat from the right side, the better. Products on the right side are high in fat, sugar, and cholesterol. If we overindulge in these foods, we must adjust elsewhere in the diet. A little hollandaise sauce on our salmon should mean no butter on the baked potato!

Food Selection Chart

BEST SELECTION	SELECTION TO LIMIT
Meat	
Lean cuts; veal	Fatty cuts; spareribs; hot dogs; bacon; sausage; luncheon meats; organ meats; canned meats.
Fish	
Lean fish: Halibut, perch, seabass, shark, snapper, tuna, etc.	Sardines, mackerel, herring, and other fatty fish.
Shellfish	
Abalone, crabs, clams, scallops	Shrimp
Poultry	
Poultry breast (skinned)	Dark meat, skin; goose, duck
Dairy Products	
Nonfat milk; buttermilk (1% fat); nonfat Yogurt; low-fat cheeses: hoop, farmers, Sapsago, mozzarella; uncreamed cottage cheese	Whole and low-fat milk; chocolate milk; sour cream; Half & Half; whipping cream; cream; non-dairy creamers; imitation milk; hard cheeses: Cheddar, American, etc.; creamed cottage cheese
Eggs	
Egg whites	Egg yolk
Fats & Oils	
Safflower oil; soft margarines	Butter, lard, bacon fat, palm oil, coconut oil, all solid fats.

BEST SELECTION	SELECTION TO LIMIT

Grains

Bread: whole grain, pita bread corn tortilla, sourdough, bran muffins

Cereal: oatmeal, grapenut, shredded wheat, buckwheat, whole oats.

Pasta: whole wheat, spinach other vegetable or grain base

Rice: whole grain rice, Bulgur, wild rice

Flour: whole grain, soy, potato

White breads, rolls, flour tortilla, biscuits, corn and potato chips, etc.

Commercial cereals, sugar coated, etc.

Egg noodles, processed white flour pasta.

White rice

White flour and white flour products.

Beans & Peas

All types

Nuts & Seeds

Chestnuts

All nuts and seeds

Vegetables

All fresh vegetables

Avocados, olives, canned vegetables.

Fruits

All fruits

Sweetened fruits, jams, jelly, dried fruit

Beverages

Fruit and vegetable juices unsweetened. Decaffeinated drinks, bottled H2O, Mineral water

Soft drinks, diet colas, alcoholic drinks, sweetened juices, caffeinated drinks, tap water.

Dressings, Sauces, Gravies

Low fat, sugar, and salt

High fat, sugar and salt

Desserts

Fruits

Ice cream, candy, pastry, puddings, honey, sugar, etc.

FOOD SELECTION SUGGESTIONS

Meats:	Eat less meat. Substitute fish and poultry breast.
Fish:	Avoid fatty fish and those packed in oil.
Shellfish:	Shrimp is higher in cholesterol than other shellfish.
Poultry:	Skinned breast is lowest in saturated fat and calories.
Dairy Products:	Emphasize nonfat products for calcium. Eat less cheese of all types and/or substitute for meat, fish, or poultry serving.
Eggs:	Limit your intake of egg yolks to 2 to 3 a week especially if your blood cholesterol is above 200 mgs.%. Egg whites are cholesterol free and high in protein.
Fats & Oils:	Safflower oil is highest in polyunsaturated fat and the essential fatty acid linoleic acid. Avoid animal fats which are high in saturated fat. Use all oils and fats in moderation. Avoid fried and deep fried foods.
Grains:	Choose whole grain breads, cereals, pastas, rice, and flour for high nutrient balance and fiber. Avoid highly processed white flour products that are high in fat and sugar and low in fiber.
Beans & Peas:	Excellent vegetable protein. Combine with grains. Avoid processed bean and pea dishes with added fat, salt, and sugar.
Nuts & Seeds:	High in fat but nutritious. Limit amount for less total fat intake.
Vegetables:	Use steamed and raw. Avocadoes and olives are very high in fat.
Fruits:	Avoid concentrated dishes with added sugar.
Beverages:	Use natural, unsweetened juices.
Dressings, Sauces, & Gravies:	Be aware of fat, sugar, salt, and calorie content.
Desserts:	Limit your intake of high-fat and sugar desserts. Use fruit more often.

Converting Grams into Calories

Throughout the book I have referred to the number of calories in food or the number of calories in each of the main nutrients. For example, we say that 81 calories in milk are fat or that 50% of the calories in milk are fat. This way of stating the figures has much more meaning than saying the product has 9 grams of fat. We can easily learn to convert grams into calories, which will help us in understanding product labels and enable us to compute the percentage of each nutrient in our daily diet. Computing the percentages requires keeping accurate records of the food we eat (using a calorie-and-gram counter). This technique is very educational and creates a real awareness of actual nutrient intake. If we suggest that your diet should consist of no more than 20% fat, this technique can allow you to compute your intake for a few days and determine an average percentage. Reading labels will become truly useful. When we can do our own conversions, we will know the facts about product content and will not have to rely on misleading advertisements for our information.

Food labels list the protein, fat, and carbohydrates in grams. These grams can be converted into calories using the following table:

1 gram fat	=	9 calories
1 gram protein	=	4 calories
1 gram carbohydrate	=	4 calories

If we convert the grams to calories for each nutrient, the total should be approximately equal to the amount of total calories in the food. Let's use milk as an example. One cup of whole milk has 160 calories, 9 grams of protein, 12 grams of carbohydrate, and 9 grams of fat.

9 grams of protein × 4	=	36 protein calories
12 grams of carbohydrate × 4	=	48 carbohydrate calories
9 grams of fat × 9	=	81 fat calories
		164 calories

Converting Calories
to Percentages

To convert these numbers to percentages, we simply divide the total number of calories into the calories for each nutrient. In the example for milk:

$$\frac{36}{160} = .22 = 22\% \text{ protein}$$

$$\frac{48}{160} = .30 = 30\% \text{ carbohydrate}$$

$$\frac{81}{160} = .50 = 50\% \text{ fat}$$

This gives us a clearer picture of what we are really eating. In the case of whole milk, we can now see that it's half fat. Knowing that fat intake should be limited, we can conclude that whole milk is a good product to avoid.

Everyone should take the time to record all the food eaten for one full day, then apply the formula described above to determine the percentage of each nutrient being consumed. In this way we can identify specific foods to reduce or increase to improve our diet.

EXAMPLE OF CALORIES
AND PERCENTAGES

Many foods now contain "nutritional information" on the label. This is usually listed in grams. Let's convert the data on a cracker label:

AK-MAK Sesame Crackers*

1 oz.:

Protein	4.64 grams
Fat	2.33 grams

*A nutritious cracker made from whole-grain wheat and sold in health-food stores. Much better than most commercial crackers, which are higher in fat and refined sugar.

185

AK-MAK (continued)

Carbohydrates   18.86 grams
Calories   117

$4.64 \times 4 = 20$ calories $\div 117 = 17\%$ Protein
$2.33 \times 9 = 21$ calories $\div 117 = 18\%$ Fat
$18.86 \times 4 = 76$ calories $\div 117 = 65\%$ Carbohydrate

Dry Roasted Peanuts (no oils or cholesterol added)
1 oz.:

Protein   7 grams
Fat   14 grams
Carbohydrate   6 grams
Calories   180

Protein   7 grams $\times 4 =$ 28 calories $\div 180 = 16\%$
Fat   14 grams $\times 9 = 126$ calories $\div 180 = 70\%$
Carbohydrates 6 grams $\times 4 =$ 24 calories $\div 180 = 14\%$

This handful of peanuts derives 70% of its calories from fat. If we eat an 8-ounce bottle of peanuts we are consuming 1,440 calories—almost an entire day's allowance!

Food Selection for Athletes

It's been stated before that physically active people should eat the same diet as "normal" people with the exception of increasing calories. This concept has some basic flaws. First, the athlete will require more calories, but it is best that these extra calories come from complex carbohydrates. Secondly, rather than athletes eating like everyone else it would be better if everyone else ate like athletes! It would be better if we all ate more complex carbohydrates and got a little exercise instead of eating the high-fat diet that is common in the United States.

For the athlete, the main function of the high-carbohydrate diet is to ensure that adequate stores of carbohydrates will be available during activity. As we have shown, depletion of carbohydrate reserves is the limiting nutritional factor in performance. Although we cannot place an exact value on their importance in specific situations, we do know that as the duration and intensity of the activity increases, energy reserves become more important. For example, the likelihood of energy depletion is greater in a marathon (an event of long duration and low intensity) than in a short sprint (an event of high intensity and short duration).

This does not mean that athletes involved in high-intensity activities can ignore carbohydrates. Any activity, especially if it is repeated over a period of time, requires available glucose. A weight-lifting match, which extends over several consecutive days, requires an adequate reserve of carbohydrates for top performance. The energy must come from "stored" reserves that are derived from a regular high-carbohydrate diet. If an athlete is not emphasizing carbohydrates in his or her diet, then the emphasis must be on fats and proteins, which will severely limit performance. All athletes should eat a basic diet high in the clean-burning natural carbohydrates found in plant foods. At least 65% of their daily calories should be derived from natural carbohydrates. The following chart shows desirable carbohydrate balances for different sports:

THE BASIC DIET FOR EACH SPORT

Low Duration and High Intensity
65% of total calories: Carbohydrate
15% of total calories: Protein
20% of total calories: Fat
Weight training, sprints, jumping and throwing events, football.

Moderate Duration and High Intensity
70% of total calories: Carbohydrate
12% of total calories: Protein
18% of total calories: Fat
Most sports: wrestling, middle-distance running, swimming, rowing, gymnastics, tennis.

Endurance Sports

80% of total calories: Carbohydrate
10% of total calories: Protein
10% of total calories: Fat

Marathon, cycling, distance swimming, cross-country skiing, hiking, triathlon.

Food Selection for Performance

CALORIE NEEDS

The dietary recommendations given throughout this book are ideal for athletes. Since the athlete is expending energy at a higher rate than the average person, he or she will require more calories. These additional calories should come from natural carbohydrates, not from protein, fat, or refined sugar. As a general rule, training of low intensity and duration will require the addition of from 200 to 500 calories per hour. Higher intensity and endurance training requires as many as 900 extra calories per hour (of exercise). This additional requirement will be met instinctively by the appetite, but the athlete must be sure to choose a good fuel source for this extra food.

SELECTING FOODS FROM THE MAJOR
NUTRIENT SOURCES FOR ATHLETIC PERFORMANCE

I. GOOD CARBOHYDRATE SOURCES

A. Whole Grains

Breads, pita breads, cereals, flours, pasta (spaghetti, macaroni, etc.), rice (brown) and corn tortillas

B. Legumes*

Beans (lima, garbanzo, black, pinto, etc.), peas, lentils

C. Fruits

All fruits eaten in their whole state are excellent carbohydrate sources. Eat the ones you enjoy within your caloric limit. Bananas and oranges are two fruits suggested for any athlete's diet.

D. Vegetables

Potatoes, corn, all other vegetables eaten raw (in salads) or steamed

II. PROTEIN SOURCES

A. Animal Sources

Meats, fish, poultry, dairy products (milk, yogurt, cheese, eggs)

B. Plant Sources

Legumes, rice, corn, whole grains

C. Examples of good plant combinations

Cereal and legumes
Wheat bread and cheese
Beans, rice, and corn
Rice and peas

---

*Excellent protein substitutes for some of your animal protein

Limit intake of animal protein to 20% of daily protein needs. All of the plant food in the diet contributes some protein. Those mentioned in II, especially legumes, are good sources. We can choose to get more protein from animal sources, but only a small amount of animal protein is required to meet nutritional needs, and animal products are high in fat. Only 3 ounces of meat, fish, and poultry will supply 21 grams of protein. Since plant foods also supply protein, it does not take many animal products to meet our needs.

FAT SOURCES

A diet selected from the carbohydrates and proteins listed on the table will ensure an adequate intake of essential fatty acids (for example, linoleic acid). Small amounts of the following are high in linoleic acid:

Wheat germ
Nuts and seeds
Safflower oil

Contrary to advice given by some well-intentioned nutritionists, do not meet your increased calorie requirements by eating high-calorie foods which are rich in fat. They reduce performance and contribute to cardiovascular disease.

DIET PLANNING

No daily menu guide is listed here, because each person should select food from the different groups shown on the basis of personal likes and dislikes. For many young athletes, this will involve some radical changes from their normal eating pattern. Eating more cereals and fruit for breakfast and eliminating ham and eggs, substituting fish and chicken for greasy meats and legumes and grains for animal protein, and eating more potatoes, rice, corn, and other vegetables will be a radical adjustment for most athletes. The benefits in improved performance and well-being will more than outweigh the inconvenience of making these positive nutritional changes.

AVOID REFINED SUGAR PRODUCTS

Nutritionists have caused most of the confusion regarding refined sugar. Because sugar is a carbohydrate, it is assumed that there is no difference between the sugar in potatoes and that in a cola. This would mean that it doesn't matter what the carbohydrate source is. One popular book about nutrition and athletes goes so far as to say that additional carbohydrates to build glycogen reserves can be obtained from a quart of Kool-Aid and a bag of jelly beans daily. Tell that to an athlete and that's all he'll eat!

Anyone, especially an active athlete, can tolerate a small amount of sweets in the diet; but when we condone the use of junk food in any form, we lend support to its proliferation. Active athletes, especially endurance athletes, can tolerate more sugar in their diet due to their higher energy expenditure, but they will still be wise to limit their intake to about 10% of their total calories. As we will see in the chapter on eating before competition, too much sugar can wipe out weeks of training.

Questions and Answers

Q: *You really come down on the food industry for not selling nuritious foods. Even the sweets must contribute something worthwhile to the diet—don't they?*
A: In advertising, it is implied that these products make a contribution to health and should play a significant role in your daily diet. You can be very healthy without most of these products. The following statement by G. Michael Hostage, President of I.T.T. Continental Baking (*Los Angeles Times,* December 9, 1980) probably best describes what food manufacturers think of their own products: "Hostess Twinkies and cupcakes are snack foods. We'd be the last to claim, I think, that anyone should eat these food products in order to get any specific diet or health value, but on the other hand, they're not bad to eat. They're 'fun foods.' They're eaten because they're simply pleasurable."

Q: *What's wrong with eating them? They are pleasurable.*
A: I've yet to see an advertisement for junk food that suggests that the product didn't contribute to health and should only be eaten occasionally. I see nothing wrong with an occasional sweet. Just don't make them part of your regular eating pattern. The more junk calories you eat, the less nutritious calories you can eat without being overweight or suffering malnutrition.

Q: *I've heard nutritionists state that fast foods aren't all that bad and in fact are well balanced.*
A: Dr. Jean Mayer, a leading nutritionists, has stated that "The typical McDonald's meal of a hamburger, french fries, and a malt doesn't give you much nutrition. It's very low in vitamins B and

C, but very high in saturated fats. It's typical of the diet that raises the cholesterol count and leads to heart disease."

Q: *Should I avoid all fast foods?*
A: If you can, yes. The fewer of them you eat the better. Assuming that the rest of your diet is adequate, a fast-food meal now and then does no harm. Its main faults are that it's high in calories, high in protein, and high in saturated fat. Fast foods, as a regular diet, are the training menu for those seeking the ultimate in heart disease.

Q: *Is there anything else bad about fast foods?*
A: Yes. Many fast foods are high in salt and low in fiber. The sad thing is that so many young people are being brought up with fast foods as a major part of their daily diet. They will be the heart attack victims of the year 2000!

Q: *Do people really eat at fast-food chains that much?*
A: *Nation's Restaurant News* states that by 1989 one-half of the food dollar spent in America will be spent on food away from home. Since fast foods are the least expensive foods to eat away from home, they corner most of the market.

Q: *Is a vegetarian diet the best diet?*
A: Compared to the typical American diet, a vegetarian diet is much healthier. A common mistake many vegetarians make is substituting high-fat dairy products for meat. They also tend to use too many high-fat plant products such as oils, soybeans, avocados, and olives. By following this type of vegetarian diet they end up with a diet just as high in fats and cholesterol as the typical American diet.

Q: *How can you expect me to eat cereal for breakfast every morning after living with eggs for twenty years?*
A: I don't expect anything from you! It's your body—you will have to make the decisions based on how important you think it is to your health. Most people find that gradually substituting cereal at breakfast and cutting back on eggs, bacon, and ham is an easy way to "wean" themselves from eating too much fat and cholesterol.

Q: *Wouldn't it be easier to list a 14-day meal plan so that I don't have to make each selection?*
A: It would be easier for me. I'd list all the foods I like. It probably wouldn't help you at all! What if I listed halibut and long-grain rice most of the time and you hated them? If *you* make your own selection, you might eat turkey breast and baked potatoes instead, which is just as good as my fish and rice.

Q: *I'm concerned about the amount of protein in my diet. Can I eat more than you suggest?*
A: Yes. But keep in mind that it doesn't take much animal protein to overdo it. If your total need is 50 grams a day you can eat more. But try to stay under 90 grams, and eat that much only if you're exceptionally big and have a high percentage of lean muscle mass.

Q: *Under meats you listed my favorite, spareribs, under the heading "Selections to Limit." Can't I eat them anymore?*
A: Think twice! Save them for a special occasion. In time you may learn to go without them. Spareribs are very high in saturated fats and calories. They're a main staple of the heart attack candidate's diet.

Q: *Can I eat a lot of the cheeses listed, such as mozzarella and sapsago?*
A: No. Even low-fat cheese is still over 50% fat and high in cholesterol. Consider your total daily intake of fat and cholesterol when eating cheese. Hoop cheese is fine, but don't expect it to taste like cheddar!

Q: *Are pizzas out?*
A: No. Just eat them occasionally. When you do, be sure that the rest of your diet that day is fat- and cholesterol-free. You will probably get more than your limit of these in that one pizza meal!

Q: *Why should I limit soybeans? I thought they were a good substitute for meat.*
A: They are, but they're also 30% fat. If your soybean intake becomes excessive, your total fat intake could go too high.

Q: *You mentioned corn tortillas as being better than flour tortillas. Why?*
A: Flour tortillas are usually made from white flour and contain added fat. Corn tortillas do not.

Q: *If I select baked goods made with whole grains, honey, and no additives, am I making a better choice than if I select commercial products?*
A: Yes. But the difference is not so significant that you can eat all you want. "Natural" cookies still are high in calories, sugar (even though it's in the form of honey), and fat. Use them just like any other sweet, as a snack once in a while, not as a daily ritual!

Q: *You mention that drinking limited amounts of good wines and beer is okay.*
A: Yes. Hopefully the cost of good-quality wine and beer will keep your intake low. It's best to limit your total intake of all alcoholic beverages, but if you want to drink, stay with beer and wine and watch the calories!

Q: *What's the best way to think of your intake of meat, cheese, fish, and other animal products?*
A: Think of small portions of animal products in relationship to your total intake of food at each meal. Eat larger servings of salads, vegetables, etc. Think more in terms of 3 to 4 ounces of meat as opposed to a typical serving of 10 ounces.

Q: *What's the advantage of whole-grain brown rice over white rice?*
A: Whole-grain rice is much higher in fiber, which means it's more filling; thus, you eat less per serving. Even though enriched white rice may be higher in specific vitamins added after milling, whole-grain rice has more of the total complement of vitamins and minerals that occur naturally in unprocessed grains. What's true for whole-grain rice is also true of all whole-grain products when compared to processed foods.

Q: *You mention eating natural ice cream as opposed to the cheaper commercial ice creams sold in supermarkets. Is it healthier for you?*
A: Not really. There's still too much fat, cholesterol, and sugar, but at least it doesn't have any additives or preservatives. Again,

the high cost should help you choose to eat less. Your best bet is not to eat any ice cream, but when you do indulge, eat the better quality products and eat it less often.

Q: *Should I eat whole fruit rather than drinking fruit juice?*
A: As a rule, yes. It contains more fiber and has less sugar. If too many calories or excess sugar are a problem for you, then whole fruits are the best choice. Even diabetics can usually tolerate whole fruit, but when they drink fruit juice they experience blood sugar problems.

Q: *As a coach, I am having trouble trying to teach our athletes the importance of not overeating. What do you suggest?*
A: It's a learning process. They have to believe in you as a coach. You might try this little cause-and-effect trick. I've used it and it gets the message across: Take your "athletes" out to lunch and load them on fat and protein (a few fast burgers, fries, and malts should do the trick). Arrive back at school just in time for the afternoon workout. During practice switch to a high-intensity, exhaustive workout. In a short time your "pig-outs" will be dropping by the wayside! Suggest that they eat a light lunch the next day and repeat the workout. To their surprise, they will notice the increased stamina and strength they have obtained.

Q: *How important is rest before competition?*
A: Very important. One major weakness American athletes have is "over-training." Resting the body prior to major competition is physiologically sound. Have you ever noticed how strongly athletes come back after a mild illness? They are physiologically and psychologically ready to go. "All work and no play makes Jack a dull athlete."

Q: *What do you know about cytotoxic testing for food allergies and its affect on performance?*
A: Not much. Dr. James Braly of Optimum Health Laboratories, located in Encino, California, seems to be the strongest advocate of this concept. Dr. Braly says that most people have at least twenty or more allergies to the foods they eat. By following a rotational diet you can eliminate many of the symptoms associated with food allergy and improve your physical energy. The theory is much more complex than this simple explanation,

but it may have some value. I would suggest that you contact Dr. Braly directly or have your doctor contact him if you're interested.

Q: *What's more important—changing the diet or supplementing a diet with vitamins and minerals?*
A: Improving the diet of the athlete is more significant to improved performance than taking supplements.

Q: *You stress the need for improving the diet, yet you think an athlete should supplement with vitamins and minerals as well, why?*
A: A maintenance level of vitamin-mineral supplements will ensure a better nutritional status than diet alone will. No one can state with complete assurance that any particular person receives an adequate intake of nutrients from diet. We can assume that we do, but we can't be sure. In all probability, highly trained athletes exceed the limits of necessity in many areas. Who's to say, for instance, that 100 miles a week is the best training mileage for all marathoners? The same is true with vitamins.

Q: *I'm a football player. You recommend I eat a diet consisting of 65% carbohydrate, 15% protein, and 20% fat. Can I eat the same as a distance runner if I want?*
A: The recommendation relates to the energy needs of athletes. All athletes can eat a diet higher in carbohydrates than the amount quoted, if they wish.

Q: *Why should athletes consume oranges and bananas?*
A: Assuming that you have no problems with these fruits, it would be worthwhile to include them in your diet. They are good sources of potassium, carbohydrate, water, vitamins, and minerals.

9
FLUID REQUIREMENTS DURING EXERCISE

Water: The Essential Nutrient

Water is one of the major factors in athletic performance. Surprisingly, many athletes and coaches don't give water nearly the attention it deserves. Dehydration causes several changes in bodily functions, all of which cause fatigue and deterioration in performance. Training, diet, and talent go down the drain as the athlete loses water through heavy work and excessive sweating.

Let's look at the physiological changes that occur as the body dehydrates.

EFFECTS OF DEHYDRATION

Reduced blood volume
Drop in blood pressure
Increase in pulse rate
Decline in circulatory function
Decrease in intracellular water
Reduced energy level
Increased body temperature

GENERAL EFFECTS OF WATER LOSS ON THE ATHLETE

3% weight loss from water: impaired performance
5% weight loss from water: signs of heat exhaustion
7% weight loss from water: danger zone
10% weight loss from water: heat stroke and circulatory collapse

Highly trained athletes and those acclimatized to heat can tolerate about 4% to 5% loss before performance is significantly impaired.

Dehydration can occur in several ways. Athletes who participate in weight-controlled sports, such as wrestling, actually attempt to perform in a dehydrated state. Endurance athletes, engaged in prolonged exercise, dehydrate as the race progresses, which reduces their performance. Football players can lose large amounts of water as a result of wearing heavy equipment and/or practicing in high temperatures and humidity, which reduces the rate of heat loss from the body. In actuality, all athletes can be victims of dehydration if one or more of the following conditions is present without adequate hydration during exercise.

1. High temperature and humidity.
2. Excessive amount of clothing and equipment.
3. High intensity and duration of exercise.

Reduced Performance and Dehydration

Dehydration results in a decline of circulatory functions. All of the activities on the cellular level that produce energy require a water environment. With dehydration, the transportation of nutrients to the working muscles is reduced, elimination of waste products is slowed, oxygen supply to the working muscles is limited, and the ability of the blood to eliminate heat from the working muscles through the skin is greatly reduced. How drastically these functions are impaired depends on the amount of water lost. For most athletes, 3% water–weight-loss results in impaired performance. For a 150-pound athlete, that's a 4.5-pound water loss, a loss which commonly occurs in most training programs (for example, football, basketball, running, wrestling, swimming).

Two points should be made very clear. First, thirst is not a good indicator of water needs during training or competition. By the time an athlete reacts to thirst, it may be too late. For example, some distance runners avoid water stations early in the race when there is no thirst, then drink large quantities in the last half of the race. Unfortunately, putting the water into the stomach does not put it into the cells. These runners will not be able to replenish their cellular water in time, and dehydration will impair their overall performance. Water must be in the tissues prior to, during, and after training or competition.

The second important point is the length of time it takes to replace lost water. A water loss of 4% to 7% requires at least 24 to 36 hours for rehydration. It is not uncommon for a high school football player to lose 4% to 5% of his weight in an early season workout. Being unconditioned and overweight (excess fat), he will find his hydration rate is considerably reduced. If our football player, at 200 pounds, lost 8 pounds (4%) during the morning workout, he should not be allowed to return to the afternoon practice because he could not rehydrate his system that rapidly. To avoid this extreme loss he should consume an adequate amount of water prior to and during workout.

Wrestlers, also, frequently lose large amounts of water weight—sometimes as much as ten pounds in two days. If the wrestler weighs 150 pounds, that is a 7% loss. At that point he should be easy to defeat, even if he's the State champion! His 7% loss will enable him to step on the scale on weight, but with competition only five hours away he cannot possibly rehydrate his system rapidly enough and will perform well below his capabilities. If he's a great deal more talented than his opponent, he may slip by. Otherwise he will lose.

Forced Dehydration
for Weight Loss

Dehydrating to attain a specific weight is most common in wrestling, but also occurs in football, basketball, rowing, gymnastics, boxing, and other sports where rapid weight loss is desired. Since 60% of the weight of an average person is water, it is easy to understand the temptation to lose weight in this quick, easy way. A typical example is that of the excessively fat 260-pound football player whose coach suggested he talk to one of the wrestlers to learn how to lose weight. In short order, the wrestler divulged his secret for weight loss: starvation, saunas, and working out with two sweat suits covered by a plastic suit. They made a cute couple jogging slowly around the track. Within two weeks, the football player was down to 225 pounds. He looked and felt like he had just escaped from a prison camp! Not only could he not play football, he couldn't even hold one. This is not the way to lose weight! Dehydration is the lazy athlete's training tool.

Wrestlers are a breed unto themselves. Many prefer to go through the tortures of dehydration and starvation a few days prior to competition to make weight rather than follow a sensible diet and training program. Why? Because it doesn't take any discipline, and it works. At least wrestlers think it works. Many wrestlers, even college and world-class wrestlers, who use dehydration are successful as often as not. They step on the mat at a reduced ability level, yet perform as capably as their opponent. The coach, spectators, and even the competitors notice the fatigue and the pain of the competition, but for some reason it's balanced equally between the two. Usually the more skilled or better conditioned wrestler wins. The reason for this is obvious. His opponent probably made weight by dehydration, too! Both wrestlers are performing at less than optimum levels, which cancels out the advantage that would otherwise have been created. What if one of these wrestlers could make weight without dehydration and perform at 100% of his potential while his opponent was only performing at 70%? All the other factors being somewhat equal, the nondehydrated athlete should win.

200

An obvious analogy is that of strength. All coaches are aware of the importance of strength in performance. All other things (talent, condition, training) being equal, the stronger opponent will win. If the opponents are equal in strength, then another factor, possibly endurance, will determine the winner. Quite possibly, if they are equal in all of these factors, dehydration may make the difference. Once the serious athletes realize this, they will be able to eliminate a major weakness in American sports. The Eastern bloc countries figured it out a long time ago, but their athletes have a stronger motivation to do what they are told!

In our own wrestling program, we did not turn the heat above normal and we discouraged sweat suits. Rubbered suits are not allowed. The athlete is encouraged to lose body fat over a long period of time and to participate in aerobic activities (such as running). Teaching *self-discipline* is an important aspect of this learning process.

Electrolyte and Mineral Replacement

The most significant electrolytes are the minerals sodium chloride, potassium, and magnesium. Much has been written that suggests a need for electrolyte replacement during prolonged exercise. To date, most of the research really indicates only a need for water. The loss during heavy exercise of water and electrolytes is not equal. Water loss is much greater and therefore demands immediate attention. Even in an exhausting workout, only 6% of the salt (sodium chloride) and less than 2% of the potassium and magnesium in the body are lost. Since large amounts of water are lost, the remaining electrolytes are actually higher in concentration. The need for electrolytes and other minerals should be adequately met by the basic diet recommended in this book.

Salt is already too prevalent in the diet, and supplements in the form of potassium and magnesium pills are not adequate. Many potassium pills contain only 100 milligrams, which seems of minimal value when one considers that the typical adult diet provides between 1,500 and 3,000 milligrams. Fresh fruits and vegetables, which should be a large part of any althete's diet, are also an excellent source of potassium and magnesium. One banana or a glass of orange juice contains 1,400 milligrams of potassium. It seems evident that fresh produce can meet many of the needs of strenuous exercise and eliminate the need to use a supplement.

ELECTROLYTE REPLACEMENT DRINKS

Popular athletes and trainers often recommend electrolyte replacement drinks during competition. Professional athletes are observed drinking various drinks throughout their game to ward off dehydration, replace lost minerals, and maintain energy. Unfortunately, research does not support the claims made by the manufacturers of these products. Electrolyte loss is not significant during exhaustive exercise such as distance running, and there is even less loss during activities that last less than an hour.

The actual evidence suggests that electrolyte drinks may delay hydration. These drinks are supposed to replace lost sweat so the manufacturers have attempted to duplicate the contents of sweat (sodium chloride, potassium, magnesium). Unfortunately, diluted sweat as a drink is not too appealing to athletes, so the makers add sugar. As usual, sugar causes nothing but problems. In this case, it defeats the entire purpose of the drinks, since it slows the time it takes for the liquid to move from the stomach into the small intestine, which means that less water is being absorbed into the blood system and hydration is inhibited.

Dr. David Costill, a leader in the research of physical performance, found that the rate of gastric emptying is directly related to the amount of sugar in the drink. When water is ingested, about 60% to 70% is absorbed into the body within fifteen minutes. Highly sweetened soft drinks, on the other hand, allow only about 5% of the water to be absorbed in the same amount of time. All drinks containing sugar will leave the stomach less rapidly than water; the rate depends on their concentration. Those who feel they must use these replacement drinks should be sure to dilute them to about twice their volume. A rule of thumb is "If it tastes sweet, dilute it more." The more diluted, the better.

The Need for Carbohydrates During Exercise

By now it should be obvious that water is the major replacement nutrient needed during competition. During prolonged exercise, small amounts of carbohydrate in a diluted form may serve to replace glucose to the liver, thus reducing fatigue. This would be important only in events lasting more than one hour (such as marathon or cycling events). For events of shorter duration which involve intermittent rest such as tournaments, track meets, and swimming meets, a mildly sweetened drink between events is suggested (fruit juices, etc.). In cases where the interval is longer (1 to 2 hours), small amounts of natural carbohydrate (fruit, bread, etc.) that will be easily digested should be adequate.

The main concern should be adequate water intake, light carbohydrate intake, and assurance that the stomach will be empty during the next event. Our wrestling team was supplied with orange juice, diluted 50%, and whole oranges. During all-day tournaments they eat no other solid food. The only exceptions are those wrestlers who qualify for the finals and have three- or four-hour breaks before the next competition. A light meal of broth, bread, and fruit or other carbohydrate would be recommended in this situation, if desired.

Salt Replacement

As I've said before, the typical American diet, consisting of highly salted processed foods, is already much too high in salt. There is plenty of salt in a diet of natural foods. There is no need for more.

It is interesting to note that Rommel's troops survived the North African desert during World War II without any additional salt in their food. Many marathoners and ultramarathoners have also been found to perform quite well on a diet that limits added salt.

Sodium (salt) is found primarily in the fluid outside the cells, while potassium is found primarily in the fluid inside the cells. The intracellular fluid is very important to the chemical actions involved with energy release. When an athlete takes salt tablets, it increases the salt concentration in the extracellular fluid. By osmosis this causes water to leave the vital inner cell and pass into the extracellular fluid to equalize the pressure and dilute the added sodium. Since the need for water is inside the cells, the addition of salt actually dehydrates the tissue. During prolonged exercise a much higher proportion of water than salt is lost through perspiration. This results in a higher concentration of salt in the extracellular fluid *without* the ingestion of any additional salt. A huge amount of water loss can be sustained before salt replacement is necessary. Most athletes get plenty of salt in their normal diet before and after competition and don't need salt during the event.

RECOMMENDATION FOR WATER REPLACEMENT TO REDUCE DEHYDRATION

A. *Daily:*

Weight: The athlete should weigh in before and after training. A persistent loss of 2 pounds or more requires additional water intake.

Diet: A high-carbohydrate diet from natural foods (grains, fruits, vegetables) will aid in normal hydration and storage of water in the muscle tissues.

Liquids:

1. Water is best for hydration.
2. All liquids aid absorption and should not be restricted.
3. Drinks containing caffeine (coffee, tea, cola drinks) should be limited since they increase the loss of water through the kidneys.
4. Alcohol should be limited. It increases water loss in the same way as caffeine.

B. *Endurance Events (one hour or more):*
   *Liquids Only:** Cool drinks (50° F.) empty stomach more rapidly than warmer drinks. Water is best.
   Diluted juices (such as orange juice). If used, electrolyte drinks should be diluted to decrease the solid particles in the drink. Select drinks that are low in sugar concentration (2 grams per 100 milliliters of water).

Two hours before competition, drink about 20 ounces of water. Fifteen minutes before the event drink about 12 ounces of water.

During the Race: Small drink (6 ounces of very diluted or water) every 10–15 minutes. (Small amounts of water are frequently tolerated better than large amounts.)
Following Competition: Eat a high-carbohydrate meal with plenty of fluids to gradually replace electrolytes and glycogen.

C. *Moderate- to High-Intensity Events over a Prolonged Period (Wrestling, basketball, football, track, golf, tennis, etc.):*
   1. Breaks between events should involve water replacement.
   2. Events carried on during hot weather should include regular breaks for water replacement (every 30 minutes during football practice or sooner if the athlete so desires).
   Liquids only: Follow the same guidelines for endurance athletes with the exception that drinking is done during the break (for example, between each tennis match).

The athlete who has two hours or more between an event may eat a small amount of carbohydrates that are easily digested (bread, soup, fruit, etc.).

Questions and Answers

Q: *You suggested cool water for hydration. Doesn't that cause cramps?*
A: No. Cool is better than room temperature—but not ice cold!

Q: *What about using a diuretic for weight loss?*
A: It causes water loss as well as a depletion of potassium, which contributes to fatigue. It's also very hard on the kidneys, and excessive abuse can contribute to kidney problems later in life.

*This practice should be especially adhered to during hot weather or in high-humidity environments that increase dehydration.

Q: *I wrestle at the 134-pound class in collegiate wrestling. I usually drop the last 4 to 5 pounds by avoiding water and using the sauna. I replace this loss by drinking water after weigh-ins. Is this okay?*
A: No. You need about 24 hours to replace the amount of water lost. You are competing at less than your maximum potential.

Q: *I notice good runners skipping the water breaks in 10-kilometer runs. Why aren't they affected by avoiding water?*
A: For two reasons. First, they're in very good condition, which in itself delays dehydration; secondly, the distance is not long enough to have a negative effect. I remember running a 10-K in Hawaii where some good runners from California did the same thing. Unfortunately, the high humidity and heat common in Hawaii caused them to dehydrate in this short race, and their times were off by as much as six minutes.

Q: *I feel better when I take some sugar during long races. Isn't this worthwhile?*
A: Only if the sugar is highly diluted in water.

Q: *You mention that coffee (caffeine) might actually increase performance, and then you state that it may stimulate dehydration. Which way should I go?*
A: Since one effect cancels out the other, it doesn't much matter. Try both ways if you wish and see what's best for you. I prefer to forego coffee or any other stimulant.

Q: *Is it harmful to use a rubber suit for losing the last few pounds before weigh-ins?*
A: It means you're lazy. The benefits are more psychological than physiological. You know you didn't discipline yourself and that will be your "crutch" if you lose: "I would have beaten him, but I was fatigued from cutting weight." Sound familiar?

Q: *When should you dehydrate to lose weight?*
A: Ideally, never! If you follow a correct diet and train at a high level you should have no trouble making weight. The day of weigh-ins you can dehydrate about 1% of your body weight without too much ill effect, but that assumes no prior withholding of liquids!

Q: *Are you sure I won't lose too much salt drinking only water during a long run?*
A: Dr. George Jessup, Director of the Human Performance Laboratory at Texas A & M University, reminds us that tap water probably contains all the salt you need to sustain bodily functions.

Q: *How does alcohol increase dehydration?*
A: Alcohol blocks the hormone ADH (Anti Diuretic Hormone) which conserves water in the body.

Q: *Just how much effect does water loss have on performance?*
A: Dr. David Costill of Ball State Univeristy has shown that a water loss of 3% to 4% of your body weight by sweating can decrease your performance in a 5,000-10,000 meter run by 6% to 7%. That's a considerable reduction, especially in world-class competition. Wrestlers commonly cut that much weight through dehydration prior to weigh-ins. I would suspect that their performance is reduced just as much as that of the runners.

Q: *Wouldn't a competitor in triathlons need more than just water during competition?*
A: Water should be the number one consideration. During the cycling, which is the second leg of the triathlon, fruit and diluted juices can be used. Don't overdo the solid food intake or you may pay for it in the last leg, the crucial marathon. Find the nourishment that has the least negative effect on your body and stick with it.

Q: *In our swimming workouts, we swim over 10,000 yards. Should I take in water?*
A: Yes. I have suggested to swim coaches that they experiment with regular water intake during workouts. This can be done by placing individualized plastic containers on the deck where the swimmer can have easy access. I think you'll find quite an improvement in your level of training if you take in water about every 15 minutes while you're doing laps.

10

THE LAST SUPPER: EATING PRIOR TO COMPETITION

It has been said that what we eat prior to competition is more likely to hurt than to help.

That statement is true. In their quest for optimum performance, athletes have indulged in all kinds of unusual dietary practices. Hunger and its supposed negative relationship to energy has caused many athletes to mistakenly believe that being full is equal to having a lot of energy. Others load up with special vitamins and minerals in the belief that they will enhance the release of energy once the event starts. Common among most athletes is the awareness that carbohydrates give you energy. This is where a little knowledge can be dangerous! Since carbohydrates give you energy, athletes unwisely choose sugared candy, soft drinks, glucose, dextrose, or other concentrated sugars which go into the bloodstream rapidly. This practice got most of its support from soft drink ads that imply we all need the "quick energy" of a little sugar. It is an ill-advised practice that has ruined many weeks of training in a matter of minutes.

Athletes like to eat what the champions eat, regardless of what that might be (vitamins, dextrose, meat, etc.). Some championship performances have been turned in on diets that would seldom, if ever, be recommended by a nutritionist. Most athletes, typically enough, want to find an easy way to win. Either of the following statements could be made by a world-champion athlete, when asked what he did to break the world record.

1. "For several months prior to the race, I took daily doses of bee pollen and Vitamin B_{15}. I'm confident it made the difference."

or

2. "I've worked my butt off for five years. I train almost daily, work with weights, and really push myself to the limit. There's been a lot of pain and sacrifice, but it's all worth it."

After the first testimonial there will be a great rush on vitamin B_{15} and bee pollen. It is unlikely that there will be the same enthusiasm for harder training and sacrifice!

As you will remember, highly talented athletes often win in spite of their ignorance of dietary habits, at least for a while. But a positive diet enhances high-level performance in the long run.

The Dangers of Overeating Prior to Competition

I have yet to see an athlete starve to death on the playing field. Yet from looking at the amount of food athletes eat at pre-event meals, you would think that starvation was imminent. The energy supplied on game day comes from the carbohydrates we have stored in the form of muscle glycogen several days prior. Food eaten on game day offers a minimal energy source. At best, its main function is to ward off hunger and the feeling of weakness associated with low blood sugar. Once an athlete understands the importance of storing glycogen, he will see the importance of eating a high-carbohydrate diet during regular training. The pre-event meal should be low in calories, high in carbohydrates, and easily digestible. The athlete who chooses to "pig out" at the training table will be assured of competing with his stomach full of food, which will detract from his performance. Cramps, lassitude, and vomiting are common characteristics of eating too much. These are hardly conducive to optimum performance. When most athletes are asked after a big meal whether they feel more like relaxing and watching T.V. or more like getting into a fight, T.V. is the runaway choice. No one wants to fight on a full stomach! Competition is a fight! That slight irritability inherent in light eating is just the thing for competition. The athlete should leave the big meals for celebrating after competition.

The Effect of Concentrated Sugar Prior to Competition

Many athletes eat a candy bar or something high in sugar just before competing to give themselves quick energy. This can be a dangerous practice which can ruin weeks of training. If the high sugar intake occurs about 15 minutes or more prior to the actual event, you may find yourself down in the dumps! At first your blood sugar rises, but this rapid blood sugar increase causes an excessive amount of insulin to be released from your pancreas to take up the rapid sugar increase in the blood. This causes your blood sugar level to drop below normal, which increases fatigue and reduces performance.

Assuming that the athlete has eaten a pre-event meal at least three to four hours prior to competition, the only worthwhile substance to ingest during the last hour is water. Popular electrolyte drinks and concentrated juices not only can trigger a negative blood sugar response, but can cause the sugar to pool in the stomach, which actually reduces the absorption of water into the system. This can add to the dehydration common in endurance events.

When I refer to concentrated sugar, I mean refined sugars such as candy, soft drinks, ice cream, and pastry, as well as honey, sweet juices, etc. The key point to remember is concentration. If the meal is several hours before competition, small amounts of sugar (fruit is best) can be tolerated; but as the competition nears, eliminate sweets!

Timing the Pre-Event Meal

Emotional stress can sometimes slow the elimination of food from the intestinal tract, causing irritation. With this in mind, it is best to eat no less than three to four hours before a competition. When I was coaching wrestling, I made it a common practice for the athletes to eat a high-carbohydrate meal the night before a tournament. For most of the team members that was the last meal. Since the larger tournaments usually started in the morning, breakfast was eliminated. The athletes found that they performed much better on an empty stomach. Their nourishment during the tournament came from water and low-carbohydrate drinks. Athletes who resist this pattern, feeling they must eat something, may be allowed a very light breakfast, which they must consume prior to 6:00 A.M. After some thought, most opt to sleep in rather than drag out of bed at 5:30 A.M. They get more rest, have less time to worry, and learn a valuable nutritional lesson. Remember, athletes perform best on an empty stomach. Even being a bit hungry is more advantageous than being satisfied.

Eat Light

The final meal, in that three- to four-hour range before the event, should be kept light. Most experts suggest about 500 calories for endurance events. Since we all differ in our caloric needs, a rule of thumb is to stop before feeling full. This is not celebration, it's preparation.

Low in Fat and Protein

Fats digest very slowly, which increases the likelihood of food still being in the stomach during competition. Fried and greasy foods, especially, should be avoided. High protein (meat, fish, etc.) is associated with high fat and can further delay the elimination time. The popular steak dinner four hours prior to game time is not recommended. That steak will remain in the stomach for ten hours after it's eaten. Another very important point to remember with regard to protein is that it contributes to dehydration by eliminating water from the tissues while it is being metabolized. This should be of concern to all athletes, especially endurance athletes (who want to prevent dehydration) and those already dehydrated (in sports involving "making weight") who are attempting to hydrate their bodies.

High in Complex Carbohydrate, Low in Concentrated Sugar

Carbohydrates will be eliminated from the stomach much more rapidly than protein and fat. This will ensure adequate blood sugar levels, which prevents the hunger and weakness associated with limited food intake. Keep in mind that a correct diet several days prior to this meal is going to be the main source of energy. The carbohydrate in this meal will play a minimal role in meeting energy demands. High carbohydrate doesn't mean "all carbohydrate"! Avoiding the sugar concentrates is the best rule. I have already discussed the problems they can cause.

High in Fluids

Athletes and coaches often do not appreciate the important role water plays in optimum performance. Once dehydration occurs, it is probably too late to correct it with any hope of improving performance. There should be concern for adequate hydration starting several days prior to competition and continuing through the activity. Emphasis on carbohydrates will increase the storage of water. Each gram of carbohydrate (glycogen) stored will retain three grams of water. Sufficient liquids, including diluted fruit juice and water, should be abundant in any pre-event meal.

Personal Preference

Avoid foods that you know will cause you irritation. Using the nutritional guidelines we have described, select foods on the basis of what appeals to you. A coach should avoid requiring a "set" meal for the team. Rather, he should suggest various alternatives that are sound, yet meet the individual athlete's personal taste. Typically we think of breakfast in the morning and dinner in the evening. For the pre-event meal, the athlete should eat what he or she feels is best. Those who want breakfast at 3:00 P.M. or dinner at 10:00 A.M. should follow their preferences.

Suggestions on the types of food to select for the last meal prior to competition, are:

BREAKFAST

Cereal with skim milk and banana sliced
Wheat toast (limit the butter)
Egg (soft or poached)
Fresh fruit slices
Orange juice
Baked potato, rice, etc.

LUNCH

Breast of turkey on whole-grain bread
Fresh fruit slices
Whole juice drink
Potato salad

DINNERS

#1:

Broiled halibut
Brown rice
Corn on the cob
Mixed salad
Whole-grain rolls
Fresh juice
Fresh fruit slices

#2:

Pasta and light clam sauce
Whole-grain rolls
Fruit juice
Fresh fruit slices
Steamed vegetables
Salad

213

LIQUIDS

Skim milk (limited)
Whole fruit juices
Whole vegetable juices
Herb tea (not caffeinated)
Decaffeinated coffee
Coffee, tea (limit)

Experimenting with these adjustments in the pre-event meal will undoubtedly improve results. If the athlete takes care to avoid foods that hinder performance rather than searching for magic foods and supplements that will spell stardom, he or she will be on the right track for success.

Questions and Answers

Q: *I worry that if I don't eat enough at the pre-event meal I'll be hungry, which will reduce my performance.*
A: You will find that your performance and well-being during competition are improved if you eat a light meal. A hungry athlete is more likely to feel competitive than one with a full stomach.

Q: *Can I eat too little?*
A: Assuming that the meals previous to the pre-event meal were high in carbohydrates, even a very skimpy pre-game meal would not have a negative effect.

Q: *I usually give my athletes dextrose prior to competition. Is this bad?*
A: Yes. Again, if previous meals are adequate in carbohydrates, extra dextrose will not be of added value. Why put more gas in a full tank? If the dextrose causes the athletes' blood sugar to drop just prior to competition, it can actually cause fatigue.

Q: *What's wrong with bacon and eggs for a pre-event meal?*
A: It's a poor choice. You may get by in low-endurance sports, but it won't help in endurance activities. It's much too low in

carbohydrates, too high in fat, which can interfere with oxygen reaching the cells, and it digests slowly, which means you may compete with it in your stomach and become nauseous.

Q: *You mentioned that each gram of stored carbohydrate stores three grams of water. Doesn't that add weight?*
A: Only a minimal amount of essential water is added. It helps in the chemical conversion of glycogen to energy and helps to delay dehydration. Don't avoid carbohydrates in the misguided belief that they add body weight.

Q: *Should I take my vitamins and minerals with my pre-game meal?*
A: Don't think of supplements as having a direct effect on performance, especially on the day of competition. It's possible they could even hinder performance if taken too close to competition. Niacin, for example, may contribute to fatigue in endurance events by blocking the use of free fatty acids and thus increase the use of glycogen, which is in limited supply. I would not take your supplements with your pre-game meal.

Q: *Doesn't sugar boost your blood sugar level if you take it just before (within 5 minutes of) competition?*
A: Yes. This may eliminate the negative low blood sugar effect, since the blood insulin is shut down during exercise. That doesn't mean it's going to increase your performance, though. It only means it may not hurt it. Again, I would suggest you avoid anything but water within the last hour prior to competition.

INDEX